Ernst Schering Research Foundation Workshop 8
Health Care 2010

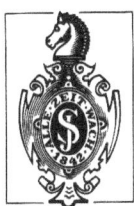

Ernst Schering Research Foundation Workshop

*Editors:* Günter Stock
Ursula-F. Habenicht

*Vol. 3*
Excitatory Amino Acids and Second Messenger Systems
*Editors:* V. I. Teichberg, L. Turski

*Vol. 4*
Spermatogenesis – Fertilization – Contraception
*Editors:* E. Nieschlag, U.-F. Habenicht

*Vol. 5*
Sex Steroids and the Cardiovascular System
*Editors:* P. Ramwell, G. Rubanyi, E. Schillinger

*Vol. 6*
Transgenic Animals as Model Systems for Human Diseases
*Editors:* E. F. Wagner, F. Theuring

*Vol. 7*
Basic Mechanisms Controlling Term and Preterm Birth
*Editors:* K. Chwalisz, R. E. Garfield

*Vol. 8*
Health Care 2010
*Editors:* C. Bezold, K. Knabner

*Vol. 9*
Sex Steroids and Bone
*Editors:* R. Ziegler, J. Pfeilschifter, M. Bräutigam

Ernst Schering Research Foundation
Workshop 8

# Health Care 2010

Health Care Delivery, Therapies
and the Pharmaceutical Industries

C. Bezold, K. Knabner,
Editors

With 15 Figures

Springer-Verlag Berlin Heidelberg GmbH

ISBN 978-3-662-03048-6    ISBN 978-3-662-03046-2 (eBook)
DOI 10.1007/978-3-662-03046-2

Typesetting: Data conversion by Springer-Verlag

21/3130–5 4 3 2 1 0 – Printed on acid-free paper

# *Foreword*

This special workshop organized by the Schering Research Foundation addressed fundamental issues facing health care and the pharmaceutical industry. It provided an opportunity to explore not future experiments but rather possible future scenarios.

Schering considers itself to be a company driven by technical progress, which in the best sense means research driven. We have had to realize, however, that the health care system is no longer – indeed, probably never has been – driven exclusively by technical progress, by progress in science. Rather, it is heavily influenced by cost constraints (such as public budget limitations), paradigm shifts, and the harmonization of Europe and the Triad. Yet we do not know for certain what directions change will take. This workshop gave us a chance to explore the uncertain future and the threats and opportunities it poses for Schering. We examined Schering strategies and how effective they are likely to be under various future conditions.

We felt it was important to acknowledge in our strategic considerations not only progress in medicine, not only the fact that medical science is a truly international science that demands and requires globalization of all our efforts. We also included the bureaucratic, the public conditions, which will to a large extent determine the marketplace by the time our compounds – with development times of 10-13 years – will finally be available.

It is remarkable that the pharmaceutical industry does indeed manage to consider these long-term goals and long-term commitments during drug development. But I was not really aware of serious attempts, at least in Europe, to properly take into account health politics, legal aspects, and other nonscientific parameters of the market that may be expected in the year 2000 and beyond.

The workshop had several goals:

- It aimed to improve our skills for thinking about the future and make us aware of the conditions of the marketplace in the year 2000 and beyond. Many governments and other bodies involved in the health care system have either issued clear proposals or have talked about how they would like to control, how they would like to structure, the health care system in the next century. So it is important to at least try to get hold of those ideas.
- It tried to enhance our imagination and creativity in considering our strategic options. Awareness creates in most cases interest, and interest encourages, in most cases, action. So one of the hoped-for outcomes of the workshop was to elaborate on the results and take them as a starting point for our own activities.
- It was designed to give the management at Schering some training in scenario techniques – a powerful tool for exploring the future in the face of uncertainty. In addition, careful consideration of the future helps us to analyze the present more prudently. Detailed analysis of the present and better understanding of trends that are already under way were the most concrete outcomes we expected from this meeting.

The workshop was also designed to leave a collection of insights which are available to the wider health and pharmaceutical community through this book.

Sometimes, looking into the future through alternative scenarios and then looking backwards at the present and noting the differences is the only way to get a bird's eye view of what is going on, what is being neglected, what is currently being overestimated, and what is being misinterpreted among all the items we manage to analyze properly. Another way of taking such a look from the distance is of course the more traditional and the one almost unconsciously used: to analyze the past carefully and then look from the past into the present and try to understand what has taken place. Yet judging the present from the past always exposes all the mistakes that we have made. So elements of excuse, of reinterpretation, of old thinking invariably cloud the picture. Looking back from the future is free of such mistakes. It is ultimately free of responsibility, because responsibility has yet to be allocated.

We asked Dr. Clement Bezold, Executive Director of the Institute for Alternative Futures (IAF), to work with us in this project. We also invited leading experts on health care and pharmaceuticals from Europe, the United States, and Japan to help us understand the changing environment for our company.

Dr. Bezold is a leading futurist who specializes in health care. He founded the IAF with Alvin Toffler to assist governments and communities to look ahead more effectively. He is currently working with the World Health Organization and the Pan American Health Organization in developing their health futures capacity.

He is also the President of Alternative Futures Associates (AFA), the private consulting arm of IAF. Through AFA he works with the largest hospital companies in the United States and the leading pharmaceutical firms there and in Europe. In addition, he works with the leading U.S. and European telephone and communication companies.

We used the scenarios to explore what might happen – the plausible future. We also discussed what we want to create – our vision for Schering.

The present is challenge enough. The future will be even more challenging. This kind of scenario workshop helped us learn more about the health care system we are living in, we are working in, and we are making money in, and it helped us understand better the trends that will be affecting this system. It will help readers of this book, beyond Schering, to similarly understand the promise and the challenges of the early twenty-first century.

*G. Stock*

# Table of Contents

1   Health Care Information Systems in 2010:
Implications for the Pharmaceutical Industry
*Jonathan C. Peck and Robert L. Olson* . . . . . . . . . . .   1

2   2010: Culmination or Continuum?
*Willis B. Goldbeck* . . . . . . . . . . . . . . . . . . . . . 29

3   The Future of Pharmaceutical Therapy and Regulation
*Louis Lasagna* . . . . . . . . . . . . . . . . . . . . . . . 41

4   The Pharmaceutical Industry in 2010
*Barrie G. James* . . . . . . . . . . . . . . . . . . . . . . 49

5   Pharmaceuticals and Health Care in Japan Through 2010
*Yoshio Yano* . . . . . . . . . . . . . . . . . . . . . . . . 67

6   The Environment for the Pharmaceutical Industry
Through 2010 in Europe, the United States, and Japan:
Alternative Futures
*Alternative Future Associates*
*in Cooperation with Schering AG* . . . . . . . . . . . . . 89

7   Workshop Summary: Change in a Challenging Future
*Clement Bezold and Linda Starke* . . . . . . . . . . . . . 105

Subject Index . . . . . . . . . . . . . . . . . . . . . . . . 115

# List of Contributors

*Bezold, Clement*
Alternative Future Associates, 108 North Alfred Street,
Alexandria, Virginia 22314, U.S.A.

*Goldbeck, Willis B.*
Ministère de la Sante Publique et l'Environment, ENS/CARE Télématics,
Cité Administrative de l'Etat, Boulevard Pacheco 19, Bte 5 Bur 711,
1010 Bruxelles, Belgium

*James, Barrie G.*
Pharma Strategy Consulting AG, Ob dem Hugliocker 48,
4102 Binningen-Basel, Switzerland

*Lasagna, Louis*
Center for the Study of Drug Development, Tufts University,
192 South Street, Suite 550, Boston, Massachusetts 02111, USA

*Olson Robert L.*
Alternative Future Associates, 108 North Alfred Street,
Alexandria, Virginia 22314, U.S.A.

*Peck, Jonathan*
Alternative Future Associates, 108 North Alfred Street,
Alexandria, Virginia 22314, U.S.A.

*Starke, Linda*
Alternative Future Associates, 108 North Alfred Street,
Alexandria, Virginia 22314, U.S.A.

*Yano, Yoshio*
International Pharma Consulting, 19-11-102 Kamiyamacho, Shibuya-ku,
Tokyo 150, Japan

# 1 Health Care Information Systems in 2010: Implications for the Pharmaceutical Industry

Jonathan C. Peck and Robert L. Olson

## Introduction

The information revolution in health care has only just begun, but already health care companies that fail to recognize the scope of change place themselves at risk. The push of technological developments and the pull of desired applications will lead the United States, Europe, and Japan to refashion health information systems. Companies in each of these markets that join the race to add value to the growing health information network will reap commensurate rewards.

Other companies will try to defend eroding positions, failing to recognize that opportunity has moved elsewhere. This chapter provides forecasts that can guide corporate decision makers to new opportunities. These opportunities are in hand because of "a new trend toward fusion of industrial sectors" (MITI 1987) that will combine the information and health care sectors in the global economy.

Alternative Futures Associates forecasts that this fusion will occur as three health information explosions detonate during the period that began in 1980 and will continue through 2010. These information eruptions will blow open new channels for data flows, sweeping aside old systems and creating phenomenal growth for companies positioned to capitalize on change.

## Explosion 1 – Automation of Inpatient Information

In the 1980s, large aggregations of data on health care costs became
feasible. In 1983 legislation in the United States mandated the use of
diagnostic-related groups, driving hospitals to place mainframe computers in their medical record departments. Computer software and
hardware sales grew spectacularly, attracting major companies, such as
3 M, to enter the field.

In the 1990s, leaders in medical informatics expect a fully automated
patient record to systematically support learning about health and illness
(Dick and Steen 1991; Foresight Seminar 1992), and political support is
forthcoming (Sullivan 1992). Quality of care and cost-effectiveness
research will also reshape data collection during this decade (Foresight
Seminar 1991a).

After 2000, information systems will integrate inpatient and outpatient care data. Many of these systems will likely follow the pattern
established in adverse drug reporting – moving from national to international data bases.

## Explosion 2 – Automation of Physician Practices

In the 1980s, physicians began to use computers for billing, but only
"hackers" were able to use computers in clinical practice. Medical
students grew accustomed to computer searches through large databases, but few practicing physicians could take the time – which ex-
plains the failure of such projects as the American Medical Association
(AMA) database service for physicians. Commercial ventures to provide group practices with computers for clinical use also failed during
the 1980s.

In the 1990s, the cost of computing power will decline sufficiently to
give physicians an ample platform for complex software designed to
make clinical applications much easier to use (Bezold and Olson 1986;
Olson and Bezold 1990). As a result, more information will be gathered
for outpatient care by an increasing number of public and private interests.

Point-of-sale data will be provided by pharmacies through prospective drug utilization review (DUR) programs (Foresight Seminar 1992).

Already, computerized systems can provide drug information in pharmacies and can alert physicians at low cost (Lipton and Bird 1991; Reindenberg 1991). Managed-care organizations will integrate outpatient service records with inpatient records.

Initial use of computers in physician practices will be for relatively mundane tasks (e.g., pop-up screens with laboratory results) that save time, allowing doctors to see more patients. Computers will later incorporate more sophisticated expert systems (software programs that provide the decision-making thought processes of experts in different domains) to assist or provide quality control for diagnosis and treatment decisions. Physicians will receive information on drugs electronically from manufacturers. The value of the information will grow significantly in relation to the value of the pharmaceuticals (Marketletter 1992).

After 2000, information networks will expand to incorporate physician systems as nodes that both send and receive information (Peck and Rabin 1989). Many of these networks will be global.

## Explosion 3 – Automation of Homes

In the 1980s, personal computers (PCs) and hardware for electronic games penetrated the consumer market in the United States, Europe, and Japan, but brought no significant applications for health. Yet significant demand for health information was visible in the enormous market for books and magazines on health (Bezold et al. 1986).

In the 1990s, health software is now being used by consumers to learn more about health and illness. Many of the programs will help patients monitor disease progression and functional capacity. By the end of the decade, many homes will also be linked into medical networks and will be sending data to providers and information vendors (Olson et al. 1992).

After 2000, homes will routinely be linked into health system networks, which will provide software and a variety of electronic services that will augment or displace current health care.

Evidence for these explosions remains incomplete. Yet companies seeking advantage from change in health systems cannot afford to ignore the indicators that exist. The patterns of change identified in this chapter can be used to reveal emerging opportunities in the medical marketplace. The logic underlying much of the change forecast here can be found in broad societal trends as well as in emerging technical capacities.

## Societal Trends

The broad sweep of change affecting the markets of Europe, the United States, and Japan can best be seen as a transition from industrial-based to information-based economies (Toffler 1990). This transition is marked by new rules, organizational structures, and relationships (Toffler 1980) that are now visible in health care systems.

*Decentralization*, for example, is moving more of health care out of factory-like environments such as hospitals and nursing homes. Health care has just begun the shift into outpatient and home-care settings; information technologies can drive this trend much further.

*Customization* creates growing demand for scientific approaches to the "art" of medicine, that is, the capacity to recognize and account for individual differences in therapeutic decision making. Information systems will empower greater customization to account for genetics and life-style. This additional information will in turn drive the demand for increasing the information infrastructure.

*Disintermediation* seeks to eliminate intermediate services and give more control to consumers or end-users (Bezold et al. 1986). In health care, this trend will bring greater demand for informed self-care. It will also turn information sources into information vendors, and vice versa.

The shift to an information-based economy can only be dimly understood in the early 1990s. Certain impacts can now be seen, however, even if they are not widely recognized. Every major cost-containment effort in the United States in recent years, for example, has been based on the growing ability to convert large amounts of data into meaningful patterns of information.

Two examples reveal how new information systems in an information-based economy are likely to play a critical role in health care cost containment. Diagnostic-related groups could be mandated by Congress for Medicare in 1983 because by then mainframe computers were inexpensive enough to store and analyze the data economically. In 1990, the Omnibus Budget Reconciliation Act (OBRA 1990) made DUR programs mandatory for United States Medicaid programs beginning in January 1993. Pharmacies in the United States computerized so rapidly between 1988 and 1990 that the electronic infrastructure allowed the DUR information system to be mandated nationwide.

This relationship between cost containment and exploding information systems will be increasingly visible. In the 1990s, existing data systems will combine with emerging information systems, pushing towards knowledge-based systems. (Already, software developers are pushing idea-processing packages to replace word processing.) DUR will merge with electronic practice guidelines linked to health outcome measures (Foresight Seminar 1991b). Payers will push this step forward for cost containment. Providers will go along because it will improve quality. And patients will find that it empowers them to make their own choices.

This desire for patient empowerment represents another significant societal trend: changing values. The "GI Generation" is yielding power to a new cohort known as the baby boomers – a trend most evident in the 1992 presidential election. In place of institution-building behavior, the "boomers" have a different pattern of challenging authority and seeking information to empower individual decision making (Strauss and Howe 1991).

To date, the baby boomers have made few demands on the health care system, but when they have, the effects have been notable. Boomers have largely gone through their years of giving birth, transforming the childbirth model in the process. Where previous generations gave up authority and responsibility to health care institutions, the boomers took it back. No longer is the father out in the waiting room and the mother "out" on the table while the doctor delivers the baby. Now both parents are in the delivery room taking part not just in the delivery, but in decision making.

A similar pattern can be seen among the population of AIDS patients, who represent another group of baby boomers who have created new demands on the health care system. AIDS activists in the United States have become remarkably well informed and extremely effective in challenging health care institutions and authorities. Patients with AIDS have made it very clear to the United States Food and Drug Administration (FDA) and to health care providers that they want to make their own choices regarding health care.

AIDS activists have already had a major impact on FDA regulations for new drug development. Continued activism will be directed towards opening clinical trials to gather more extensive data from community-practice settings (Foresight Seminar 1989). This activism fits the pattern established at a young age by the baby boomers. It creates an important barrier to the potential for emerging information systems to favor the interests of larger institutions by discriminating against individuals, a possibilty that is a real fear for AIDS patients (Peck and Bezold 1992).

The value orientation of the GI generation that has held power for the past 32 years created demand for information technologies that served institional interests. The value shift now under way may be symbolized by the demand for a different kind of computer that surprised the mainstay computer industry in the 1980s. It was not mainframe computers – perhaps the best symbol for a technology designed to serve large institutions – that dominated the decade. It was the PC which empowered individuals and began to transform large institutions.

As we look ahead to the technological developments that are reshaping the health care marketplace of the 1990s, it is important to keep in mind that it is not just the technologies that need to be considered. Larger societal trends will define how the technologies will be used.

## Technological Paradigm Shift

The most important thing to understand about the basic information technologies that underlie health information systems is that they are not just improving rapidly, they are going through a "paradigm shift." A technological paradigm shift is a change to a fundamentally different approach with new kinds of technology, new capabilities, new organizational arrangements, and new ways of thinking (Olson 1991).

Looked at from the point of view of telecommunications, the paradigm shift taking place today involves three enormous, interconnected changes. First, the "analog empire" of traditional analog-based telephone networks is collapsing, being replaced by what Microsoft's founder Bill Gates calls "a new digital world order." Digital switching and the "digitization of data" of all kinds allow communication networks to carry voice, data, text, images, and video signals simultaneously. Digitized data can also be rearranged, combined, and manipulated with ease, making possible a new domain of true "multimedia" communication (Coates 1992).

Second, the new digital world order is merging telecommunications with computing and video (Gilder 1991). Computers everywhere can be linked. What used to be called telephones and television sets are becoming computer terminals, and telecommunication lines are becoming the extended circuitry of networked computers.

Third, the bandwidth or frequency span of telecommunication channels is increasing dramatically, allowing more data to be transmitted in a given amount of time. This speedup is beginning to allow a new realm of "bandwidth hungry" applications such as videophones, video teleconferencing, high-resolution image transfer, multimedia mail, and multimedia database access (Olson et al. 1992).

On the computing side, the "fourth paradigm" of computing is beginning to emerge. The initial paradigm was the standalone mainframe that batch-processed information for large companies, the military, and researchers. Computers improved within the context of this paradigm from World War II through the 1960s until a breakthrough occurred to the second paradigm of "time sharing" computing. There was still a central computer, but its services were shared by many subscribers, each with their own terminals. Within a decade, young computer hackers pioneered an even larger paradigm change, the invention of PCs. The spread of PCs in the 1980s turned information processing into a personal productivity tool used by every business and large numbers of individuals (Olson 1991).

Now computing is in the early stages of another fundamental shift, from the dominance of standalone PCs to a synthesis of computing and communication. The change is much larger than earlier ones because it combines dramatic improvements in computer power, miniaturization, and artificial intelligence with the enormous changes occurring in telecommunications.

To appreciate how greatly information technology will reshape the health care system, it is necessary to explore how this technological paradigm shift will unfold between now and 2010. While detailed market forecasts are impossible, the overall pattern of long-term change is already reasonably clear (Scientific American 1991). Major features of the emerging paradigm of information technology are summarized below. For those interested in a fuller discussion of technological change, more extensive forecasts are provided in the following section.

- Devices of all kinds, from telephones and TV sets to note pads and bulletin boards, will become computers or contain computers. New general-purpose "information appliances" will integrate functions now provided by telephones, PCs, TVs, video game machines, and other devices.
- Computers will become multimedia devices – processing video, high-resolution still images, and sound as well as text.
- Communication networks will become end-to-end digital soon after the end of the century. The "networking of digital networks" will evolve towards an integrated national information infrastructure.
- Large numbers of computers, information appliances, and computer-containing devices will be connected to the evolving information infrastructure. Interconnection rather than standalone devices will become the rule.
- The spread of optical fiber through the information infrastructure will create an "information superhighway system" capable of providing effectively an unlimited communication bandwidth to homes as well as businesses.
- Continued miniaturization will make it possible to put what are now called "supercomputer" levels of power in tiny integrated circuit chips. Notepad and palmtop-sized computers will proliferate everywhere, using color, high-definition, flat screens.
- Neural networks and other parallel computer architectures will make computers faster at many tasks and much better at pattern recognition, allowing dramatic improvements in speech recognition, computer vision, and many other functions.
- Graphic interfaces, pen-based computing, and speech recognition will make computers exceptionally easy to use and more truly portable than ever before. (Hand-held computers with electronic "pens" or voice input and phone links will be among the technologies most widely used by health care providers.)
- A new realm of "personal" communications will emerge rapidly with the explosive growth of cellular and personal communications systems (PCS), pocket phones, portable computers with cellular modems, and personal number calling.

- Computer/communication devices will be used by groups as readily as by individuals, with teleconferencing and new kinds of "groupware" to facilitate cooperative work and learning.
- Powerful memory chips will complement optical technologies in providing a new level of information storage capability. Before 2010, new types of storage technologies will emerge to provide super-massive desktop storage.
- New approaches to the organization of knowledge, such as hypermedia, will allow major improvements in information access and ease of learning. Hypermedia will allow users to navigate through large bodies of multimedia material, following their own interests, moving easily between overviews and detailed information, and jumping at will to visual demonstrations, simpler or more complete explanations, source materials, opposing views, related subjects, and so on.
- Expert systems will proliferate in every field, becoming more sophisticated and easier to create and use.
- Progress in artificial intelligence (AI) will begin to transform computers into more active "personal digital assistants" that can manage schedules, seek out information, and even learn from experience how to be more helpful.

## Detailed Technology Forecasts

This section describes in more detail the level of information technology capabilities that seem likely by 2010 and highlights some key developments along the way. Forecasts are set out on computer power, software, storage, input and display, and telecommunications.

These forecasts make it clear that information technology is still in an early stage of development and is evolving even faster than most analysts predicted a decade ago (Olson and Bezold 1990). In many areas, performance is increasing by 20%–50% per year, and the price for a given level of performance is decreasing at least as fast. No fundamental technical limits in sight within the next two decades would prevent this phenomenal rate of technical progress from continuing (R. Finley, personal communication). Societal factors such as sustained economic hard times, industry conflicts, or shortsighted policy making could slow the pace of change, but progress will be dramatic even in unfavorable conditions (Bezold and Olson 1986).


## Computer Power

### *Microelectronics*
The ability to squeeze more and more components onto tiny integrated circuit chips is one of the great driving forces in the overall evolution of information technology. The number of transistors that can be put on a single microchip quadruples every 3 years (Gilder 1991). In the mid-1980s, most experts believed that at most 100 million transistors could eventually be packed on a chip – more than a hundredfold improvement over the chips available at the time. They expected to reach this level around the year 2000 (Mayo 1985).

Those forecasts have been rendered obsolete by dramatic progress over the past few years in nanofabrication techniques – the ability to put down atomically thin layers of matter, producing a new realm of two-dimensional "lattice matter" that does not exist in nature. The projection of 100-million-component chips by 2000 now looks like an underestimate by a factor of two to four (Olson and Bezold 1990).

It appears possible to put a billion or even 10 billion transistors on a single chip by 2010 – a thousandfold or ten-thousandfold improvement from the mid-1980s. A billion-component chip would have the power of the central processing units (CPU) in 20 Cray 2 supercomputers (Gilder 1991).

### *Microcomputers*
With the introduction of 486-class microprocessors in the early 1990s, microcomputers are beginning to overlap the processing power of low-end mainframes (17 million instructions per second or MIPS). By 2000, Bell Communications Research forecasts that multimedia PCs more powerful than today's best SUN workstation models will be available in the price range of current TV sets (I. Dorros, personal communication). Well before 2010, super-scale integration chips will make possible "microsupercomputers," desktop and portable computers with more power than a late-1980s Cray 2 supercomputer that runs at nearly 2 billion gigaflops or floating point operations per second (Yoder 1992).

### Minicomputers and Mainframe Computers

At the start of the 1990s, clustered microprocessor designs are being used to create minicomputers more powerful than any 1980s commercial mainframes (over 500 MIPS). By 2000, minicomputers with the processing power of late 1980s supercomputers will effectively replace mainframes (R. Finley, personal communication; Hooper 1992) and by 2010, "computational utilities" will supply computer power, making differences between minis and mainframes irrelevant.

### Supercomputers

Today's large supercomputers run at 1–10 billion gigaflops per second. The High Performance Computing Initiative passed by Congress in 1991 anticipates before 2000 roughly a ten thousand times increase in supercomputer power and a ten million times increase in the transmission speed of the networks linking supercomputer users (HPCCA 1991). By the mid-1990s, the largest parallel processing supercomputers will achieve teraflops speed – over a trillion operations per second (Elmer-DeWitt 1988). By 2010, the largest supercomputers could have on the order of a billion processors and would serve as "computation power utilities" providing extra power for connected computers (D. Hillis, personal communication).

### Parallel Processing Computer Architectures

During the 1990s, parallel architectures that link small numbers of powerful processors will force computer makers to abandon conventional CPU-based mainframes. The development of "massively parallel" architectures linking large numbers of weak processors will produce even more striking improvements in computer speed. Neural networks and other massively parallel architectures will lead to dramatic advancements in computer speed, pattern recognition, machine learning, the handling of incomplete information, and the solving of problems that cannot be dealt with by applying predetermined rules or algorithms (Tank and Hopfield 1987).

By 2000, many computers will have hybrid architectures – part serial, part parallel. Neural network retina and cochlea (inner ear) chips will give some computers increasingly human-like sensory capabilities (Gilder 1989). By 2010, massive parallelism will dominate computer design.

## *Distributed Computing*

In the past, data flowed too slowly through computer networks to allow the division of computational tasks between interconnected machines. But high-speed optical fiber networks are emerging and a good deal of progress has been made in the past 4 years in agreeing on the standards and interfaces that will allow distributed computing.

Later in the 1990s, high-speed networks will allow researchers to break problems into parts that can be assigned to different computers in different locations – parallel supercomputers, serial machines, specialized processors, workstations, PCs, and so on. Networks of cooperating workstations or PCs will be able to operate at teraflop speeds right along with the most massive supercomputers (D. Hillis, personal communication). By 2010, distributed computing and the use of the largest supercomputers as computation power utilities will allow desktop computers to be "as powerful as necessary" (D. Hillis, personal communication).

## Software

### *Software Productivity*

Software production will shift rapidly during the 1990s from being mainly an "art" practiced by highly individualistic programmers to being a partially automated, mass production-like activity. Many of today's emerging automation efforts are known as computer-aided software engineering (CASE). Most software firms do not yet use CASE tools – in the United States, only 15% of all software companies have invested in them.

By 2000, CASE tools will be universally employed to assist programmers and, increasingly, to get computers themselves to generate software. Reusable standard-function software modules and very high level programming languages will make software production easier and faster (Bezold and Olson 1986).

The path of progress beyond 2000 is less clear for software than for other areas of information technology, and some analysts fear that the difficulties involved in creating ever more complex software programs will be a serious bottleneck in information technology development. Our own assessment is that by 2010 advanced software tools using massively parallel computers will abate this software bottleneck. Dynamically self-programming neural networks will also make software development less central to success for many applications (Gilder 1989).

### Parallel Languages

In the early 1990s, the use of parallel computer architectures will be slowed by the need to learn to write software in new ways. The Sigma I and Sigma II projects in Japan could help provide such learning, which would create a strong foundation for emerging programmers in Asia, Europe, and the United States.

By 2000, a new generation of programmers from different regions of the globe will find parallel programming easier and more natural than conventional programming (D. Hillis, personal communication). By 2010, computers may well be programming computers in parallel languages incomprehensible to humans.

### Expert Systems

At the beginning of the 1990s, one type of AI application, expert systems, is beginning to spread in areas as diverse as telecommunications network routing, health care, and electric power plant operation. Diagnostic programs such as the Apache system for emergency medicine are already in use in hospitals. General Physics sells a Thermal Information Program that monitors exit gas temperature and recommends steps to reduce waste. Much of the development is taking place internally to improve corporate productivity rather than as products sold in the marketplace.

By 2000, expert systems dealing with narrow domains of knowledge will proliferate into most areas of business and professional work. Broad expert systems, linking scores of narrow expert systems with a background of relevant "common sense" knowledge, will be used in areas such as health care where knowledge can be most easily codified. By 2010, self-improving expert systems will continually learn from experience.

### Flexible Information Processing

Overcoming the "brittleness" of current AI systems – their inability to respond to new situations – has emerged as a central challenge. Japan's new MITI-funded Real World Computing (RWC) Program will focus directly on this challenge of moving towards "flexible information processing." The goal is to deepen theories for "soft logic," pattern recognition, neural computing, machine learning, multivariate data analysis, and probabalistic and statistical inference, and then to unify these theories in prototype applications (Yonezawa 1992).

## *Hypermedia*

Hypermedia software that links text, sound, images and video stored on optical disks is coming into the marketplace at the start of the 1990s. During the 1990s, a great variety of hypermedia programs will be developed that allow users to pursue self-directed learning using large bodies of multimedia material. They will be able to jump at will to overviews, explanations, video demonstrations, source materials, alternative viewpoints, related topics, and the like. Hypermedia can provide layered levels of information, so that newcomers to a topic get introductory information while more knowledgeable users get more complex and detailed information. It can also be used to customize presentations of information to adapt to different learning styles, cognitive strengths, and backgrounds (Nelson 1987; Dede and Palumbo, unpublished).

By 2000, information organized in hypermedia formats will be widely used for corporate training and personal learning. Organizing information into patterns that foster both "instant expertise" on narrow topics and "accurate overviews" of large topics will be a greater focus of attention than traditional processing of text, numbers, data, and images (Larson 1992). Between the mid-1990s and 2010, "broad" hypertext systems spanning wide areas of knowledge will also become available through information networks, building towards the creation of a global knowledge access system (McAleese 1989; Nelson 1987).

## *Knowbots*

Knowbots (knowledge robots) are a developing class of AI functionalities that operate in individual computers and communication networks to search out requested types of information from electronic databases. They improve with experience at finding information that closely matches the interests of their users. Experimental knowbots have already been created in software designed at places such as the Corporation for National Research Initiatives (R. Binder, personal communication).

Knowbot technology will enter high-end business markets in the late 1990s, making possible new "narrowcasting" services such as "personalized newspapers" compiled from a variety of wire services and news feeds (Brand 1987). By 2010, low-cost knowbot technology will be starting to have revolutionary impacts on business, education, and personal learning. John Skully, CEO of Apple Computer, believes that in 50 years people will wonder how anyone ever learned effectively and kept up to date without this kind of capability.

### Language Processing

At the start of the 1990s, research on natural language processing is beginning to move out of universities and into the marketplace. Microsoft and other software firms have recently begun to make major expenditures to develop a future generation of software that will incorporate natural language processing (Gates 1990). Speech recognition of a several-thousand-word vocabulary has been available for years, but it has been expensive, speaker-dependent (the system must be "trained" to the speech of its user), and tedious (slow speech with spacing between words is required). A turning point is being reached, however, with the first low-cost, continuous speech recognition systems about to come on the market (such as Apple's Casper system).

By 2000, speaker-independent, continuous speech recognition systems will probably have vocabularies of 5000 words or more – adequate for nearly all purposes. Many computers and devices will be voice-controlled. Machine translation of written text to other languages will be "good enough" for many purposes.

By 2010, large-vocabulary continuous speech recognition will be inexpensive and ubiquitous. Machine translation will only require human review when total accuracy or stylistic beauty are needed. The phone system will provide automated simultaneous translation (Keller 1992).

### Storage

Magnetic memory remains the dominant storage medium at the start of the 1990s, but profound technical shifts are under way. Optical storage, much of it in a compact disk (CD) format, is beginning to usher in a new era of multimedia computing. Semiconductor memory is improving rapidly, with 16-MB dynamic random access memories (DRAMS) already available.

Well before 2000, optical storage will be standard on multimedia PC workstations. Gigabit memory chips will eliminate the need for mechanically rotating magnetic or optical memory in many applications. At the same time, memory requirements for storing images and video will be slashed by image compression techniques (Carlton 1991).

By 2010, magnetic memory will be largely replaced by large, nonvolatile semiconductor memories that can keep data in storage without backup power for centuries. New technologies such as frequency domain optical storage, electron beam recording, or holographic associative memory in neural networks will make massive storage available on the desktop (Olson and Bezold 1990). It is possible that molecular-scale electronics, with three-dimensional data storage in protein molecules, could begin to be commercialized by 2010. Recent experiments with genetically engineered bacteria protein suggest that the entire Library of Congress could ultimately be stored in a six-cubic-centimeter biochip (Naj 1991).

## Input and Display

### *Input*
At the start of the 1990s, the keyboard was still the dominant way people entered information into computers, but alternatives such as handwriting input are growing in importance. By 2000, pen-based computing and voice input will compete effectively with keyboards in many applications. "Physical interaction input" will also be important in some situations, such as hand movements that manipulate objects on the computer screen. By 2010, voice input will probably replace the keyboard as the primary means for people to enter information. Experimental systems will use direct nervous system control of computers (Moravec 1988).

### *Display*
The 1990s will see the development and widespread use of high-definition imaging systems, inexpensive liquid crystal flat screens that display

color pictures at video speeds, and technologies such as ferroelectric liquid crystals (FLC) that allow color video displays a meter on a side or larger (Zachary 1992). Tiny "eye screens" will appear in the market that can integrate a computer display into a viewer's visual field (Kluger 1989).

By 2000, high-definition television (HDTV) will set the standard for on-screen images. For small and mid-sized screens, flat panel displays will equal cathode rat tube (CRT) performance. Improved eye screens, combined with dramatic improvements in computer graphics, will create "magic glasses" that immerse users in realistic "artificial realities" (Moravec 1988).

By 2010, flat panel displays will probably have replaced CRTs for all uses. "Magic glasses" will be widely used and will provide three-dimensional viewing. Full-motion holographic displays will be available but expensive.

**Telecommunications**

At the start of the 1990s, digital networks are rapidly being put into place by government telecommunications and postal agencies, regulated telecommunications companies, and private firms. These networks are becoming increasingly "intelligent" and versatile, with computer control distributed among switching centers throughout the network and even at the customer end. Optical fiber is technically ready to be widely deployed into offices and homes; it is now mainly a matter of investment rates to get fiber fully into the marketplace. Mobile communication is the fastest growing segment of telecommunications: cellular technology is continuing to spread, and new personal communication systems that support pocket phones are just entering the market. Integrated Service Digital Network (ISDN) channels will become widely available during the mid-1990s, doubling the speed of telephone lines. At the same time, rapid progress in integrated circuit chips could lower the costs of image compression so that, by the late 1990s, image-oriented and video applications could be flourishing based on ISDN and conventional phone lines. Cooperation between phone and cable TV companies could also speed the transition to multimedia communications (Olson et al. 1992).

By 2000, the public-switched telecommunications networks will be nearly end-to-end digital, and multimedia integrated voice and data services will be common. Most new and refurbished wiring to offices and homes will employ optical fiber. High-capacity optical fiber networks for research and education will be in place, and dramatic progress will have occurred in the rate at which information can be sent through fiber and the distance information can travel without amplification. Direct broadcast satellites (DBS) will slash the cost of receiving information from satellites. Explosive growth in "personal communications" will be revolutionizing telephony: on nearly half of all calls, at least one party will use wireless access, and personal number calling will allow people to take their personal phone numbers with them wherever they go (A. Chynoweth, personal communication).

By 2010, optical fiber will reach a third to half of all homes in the United States and Western Europe, and even more in Japan, and a transition will be well under way to a gigabit broadband network. What researchers at Xerox Corporation's Palo Alto Research Center call ubiquitous computing will create work environments filled with inconspicuous computers connected by radio links. Common office tools – like note pads, blackboards, and Post-its – will be imbued with computer "intelligence" and the capacity to create and transmit electronic documents (Markoff 1991).

## Applications in Health

The technological developments just described provide a view of the potential of the information revolution in health care. To see it more clearly, however, it is necessary to think imaginatively about the interaction of all these developments. The combination, for example, of handwriting and voice input, color flat screen and "magic glasses" display technology, cellular modems and personal communication systems, knowbot software, and microsupercomputers the size of cigarette packs will open up radically new possibilities for fully mobile and personal access to nearly all information resources and computer-based capabilities.

To understand not only what is possible, but also what is plausible, it is important to know what public and private interests want. This section contains forecasts based upon both forecasted technology and applications that policy makers, practitioners, and consumers will seek.

## Research Tools

The amount of computing power sought for research has grown exponentially through the 1980s. The sophistication of research has increased as well in areas such as molecular biology, human genetics, neuroscience, and many other fields. The speed at which new knowledge from basic research gets translated into applications is likely to accelerate.

High-end supercomputers began to be purchased by pharmaceutical companies for complex molecular modeling in the late 1980s. Databases for clinical trials were automated in the 1980s and will soon be integrated electronically into computer-assisted new drug applications (CANDAs).

In the 1990s, clinical research data will be automated so fully that community physicians will be able to participate in clinical trials. Manufacturers will provide software for easy patient enrollment.

After 2000, distributed computing power will provide basic researchers with a capacity to model complex molecular cascades that are keys to understanding the workings of the human brain and the human genetic code. Information systems will create continuous monitoring of drug experience throughout the world. Post-marketing surveillance will replace much of the research demand for clinical trials. The distinction between research data and market data will largely disappear.

## Standardized Electronic Medical Records

Electronic medical records will record and store all patient information including patient problems, examination findings, orders submitted, test results, and treatment plans. Resistance to these enhanced medical records will persist through the early 1990s, or as long as the technology is less convenient for the physician to use than current paper forms. Privacy concerns and the potential for electronic medical records to affect current power relationships (that is, doctor to patient or doctor to payer) also could delay adoption of electronic medical records. By the mid- to late 1990s, however, the pervasiveness of powerful electronic platforms will overcome some of these difficulties.

The formats used in the early 1990s will make electronic records feel familiar to physicians now using paper records. Voice-input and output will join various touch screen and pen-based devices to encourage acceptance and enhance the use of electronic medical records.

There will continue to be competing medical record development efforts in the United States and in Europe, though coordination is likely by the mid-1990s. Japan will lag behind for cultural reasons. Information-system vendors and third-party payers will have a major role in determining what the record contains.

By 2000, many of these medical records will include a patient's "DNA fingerprint", or portions thereof. Electronic medical records will increasingly include life-style information, such as nutritional patterns, emotional states, and environmental exposures. By 2010, the primary medical record generated by providers during each encounter will be integrated with each patient's longitudinal record, which will begin while the person is in utero.

## Health Outcome Measures

Much health care goes unevaluated. The drive for outcome measures is a major effort to ensure that health care providers and therapies are evaluated systematically. Because double-blind placebo trials cannot be used to measure comparative outcomes practically, researchers have adopted survey research techniques. These methods are joined with other measures to predict the likely outcomes of a given therapy.

Major public and private programs are under way in the United States to develop and apply outcome measures. Ultimately, outcome measures will allow the comparison of the results of various health care providers and therapies. The initial public-sector applications, however, will be through the Agency for Health Care Policy and Research (AHCPR), which will evaluate the outcomes of expensive surgical procedures that are thought to be performed at unjustifiably high rates (such as hysterectomies, prostatectomies, and heart by-pass operations).

By the late 1990s, health outcome measure research will be used by the United States government to restrict payment to providers. After the year 2000, health outcome measures will converge with cost-effectiveness studies and the development of protocols to direct therapeutic selection in the United States. Europe may adopt a similar approach if there is evidence that it will provide both a cost-containment and quality assurance mechanism.

Outcome measures will also develop from the consumer/user of health care. Current consumer-based systems focus on general evaluations of consumer satisfaction with providers. These rating groups are likely to grow. As they do, and as consumers' medical records become more sophisticated, electronic, and in the consumer's possession (for example, with smartcards), it will become easier to combine measures of clinical outcomes with patient satisfaction measures.

Drug cost-effectiveness studies will be incorporated into outcome measures. These studies will become common in the 1990s, and increasingly they will include quality-of-life components in addition to cost data.

Outcome measures will identify variations in success of therapies for different subgroups in the population. This development will lead to more complexity in therapeutic decisions, whether made by human providers or by expert systems. For example, some drugs that are now viewed as "Me-too" drugs will prove to be breakthroughs for 10% of the treated population.

## Expert Systems in Clinical Practice

### Diagnostic Systems

In the 1980s, the QMR expert system at the University of Pittsburgh provided the most extensive diagnostic system, but it is primarily useful as a teaching device. Numerous programs that are less ambitious have been developed, but none are widely accepted.

In the 1990s, expert systems will become more capable of making differential diagnoses. The natural history of aging, the natural history of diseases, the genetic predispositions to disease, and the impact of current health conditions will be integrated into diagnostic algorithms. These diagnostic systems will be available in physician workstations and used for consultation and quality control.

After 2000, expert systems will produce diagnoses tailored to the biochemical uniqueness of the individual. They will be available for consumer use.

### Therapeutic Systems

In the 1990s, most expert systems will be developed as "decision support" tools for providers, giving clinical guidelines and the ability to assess the variability of care for any given patient in relation to practice standards. These support systems will suggest the appropriate work-up testing sequence and treatment patterns for specific illnesses. One example is the 3 M HELP Patient Care System that is currently on the market.

In the latter 1990s, such systems will be effectively linked to the electronic medical record and databases that will advise the practitioner on the logic and the medical literature supporting specific decisions. Appropriate educational materials will be provided directly to the patient from these systems.

After 2000, therapeutic systems may be accessed directly by patients who will be assisted by AI software as well as by healers.

### Preventive Systems

Most people in the United States will be in some form of managed care system in the 1990s. These systems will shift provider incentives towards prevention programs at a time of strong movements by consumers and employers in the direction of health promotion/prevention.

Expert systems in the mid-1990s will prompt clinicians to perform preventive health procedures, health screening tests, and timely follow-up measures. They will be linked to the consumer/home and behavioral systems described below.

## Consumer Information Systems

Consumers will have greater health information available to them at home and in a variety of settings – from the physician's office to their pharmacy. This will include:

– Sophisticated clinical advice about specific diseases

- Information on their own health conditions and normal expectations
- Access to their medical record
- Integration of their diet and exercise routines with their medical forecasts
- Access to evaluations of local providers and evaluations of various therapies
- "Health coach" systems that will provide advice for each family member that aids in shaping behavior

These systems will evolve in the late 1990s at different speeds, depending on the status of local electronic networks, providers' movement into these services, and consumers' home information systems.

## Behavior Modification (The Health Coach)

Life-style factors account for a very large part of the variation in illness in most patients. Behavioral problems also often reduce compliance with therapies. The 1990s will see more sophisticated expert systems that interact with each individual to reinforce positive, healthier behavior.

After 2000, low-cost voice input and output will allow these expert systems to "talk" with each family member at the knowledge level appropriate to that person. These "Health Coach" expert systems, backed up by the knowledge of leading specialists, will be given to people by their health care providers.

## Consumer Evaluation Systems

The 1990s will see the more effective rating of physicians and institutional providers based on results from more sophisticated medical recordkeeping, and particularly on outcome measures. Employer and insurer groups will press for systems that help them, their employees, and their customers to choose physicians on the basis of quality and cost-effectiveness.

Most major communities in the United States will have consumer-based evaluation groups by the year 2000 that will evaluate a wide range of products, services, and vendors. Among those being reviewed will be health care providers. Such services now exist in some cities, with physician ratings based primarily on customer satisfaction, including presumed outcomes. As medical records become more sophisticated, electronic, and accessible to consumers, people will be able to provide selected portions of their records to consumer organizations for aggregation.

## Medical Practice Management Systems

The 1980s saw a growing number of vendors for systems aimed at the physician practice market. In the early 1990s, vendors are working to integrate patient scheduling, billing, and internal-resource scheduling (physicians, nurses, equipment). The most successful efforts will improve physician productivity and offer a clear return on investment.

Some vendors are entering strategic alliances with health care systems. For example, the computer firm EDS and the Harvard Community Health Plan (HCHP) jointly own one of the leading-edge companies working to this integration process. HCHP will apply the results in its health maintenance organization, one of the largest in the United States. Plans include the possibility of providing members with "minitel" terminals to obtain access to the home care component of their managed care system.

## Automated Protocols

Medical practice guidelines and protocols are now being developed in various settings and they will be embedded in software used by physicians. In the 1980s, formularies were instituted in most hospitals and managed care organizations, creating limited practice guidelines for physicians. Formularies were not generally automated.

In the 1990s, formularies will be automated and made available to physicians by hospitals, managed care organizations, and other insurers. Medical protocols for treatment regimens will be developed (AMA is currently working on this with the RAND Corporation) and automated as well.

After 2000, providers will deliver care using networked protocols that are continuously updated to account for worldwide experience with therapies.

**Drug Utilization Review**

DUR programs assess data on drug use against explicit standards and introduce remedial strategies to achieve objectives such as cost reduction, detection of fraud, and improved quality of patient care. Retrospective DUR occurs by examining data on past prescribing. Prospective DUR assesses whether a prescription meets standards before the prescription is given to a patient.

In the 1980s, DUR developed in inpatient settings and extended to some outpatient care. A national prospective DUR system was mandated in the United States in 1988 in the Catastrophic Care Act, which was subsequently repealed.

Congress added DUR provisions to its Omnibus Budget Reconciliation Act of 1990 (OBRA 1990). There will be a rapid expansion in point-of-sale computers used in pharmacy practice during the early 1990s, providing data for research and commercial use. Later in the decade, data from DUR programs will be integrated with patient information from both large health care systems and physician practices.

After 2000, DUR will be integrated with data from providers (showing the medical assumptions) and data from households (showing compliance and cofactors affecting the outcomes of drug use). Information on drug utilization will displace much of the market information that is currently sold by vendors. Physician product selection will be largely shaped by DUR and formularies.

**Monitoring Systems**

In the 1980s, the use of 24-h monitors grew (such as the Holter Monitor for ECGs), and telemonitoring between physician offices and patients developed (for example, for asthma).

In the 1990s, biosensors and expanded computer capacity in homes will promote rapid growth in the use of home monitoring systems that will be linked to computers in physician offices and managed care organizations. Monitoring systems will also be designed for clinical research to accumulate information on compliance, pharmacokinetics, and pharmacodynamics.

After 2000, monitoring systems will be integral to diagnosis and treatment as well as prevention efforts. Monitors will provide information not only on biochemical changes but on behavior, environment, and bioelectric effects as well. Information systems will link consumers, providers, and payers.

## Conclusion

The physician's environment and the entire health care system will be profoundly altered by health information systems in the decades ahead, and companies that do not recognize the pattern of change may find their markets invaded by surprising new competitors. If only half the forecasts contained in this chapter prove to be accurate, health care companies will face significant challenges.

Powerful competitors have entered or soon will enter the health information arena to capture the advantages of a growing information infrastructure. Long-term competitive success for companies will depend on their ability to recognize challenges before they become critical. This ability begins with a clear vision of the future that informs strategies, operations, and tactics in the marketplace. Such a vision must encompass both the external factors discussed here and the internal strengths of companies that seek long-term success.

## References

Bezold C, Olson RL (1986) The information millennium: alternative futures. Information Industry Association Report

Bezold C, Carlson RJ, Peck JC (1986) The future of work and health. Auburn House, Dover, Massachusetts

Brand S (1987) The media lab. Penguin, Middlesex

Carlton J (1991) Chips & technologies develops a chip that permits television-style images. Wall Street Journal, January 9: B3

Coates VT (1992) The future of information technology. Ann Am Acad 522: 45–56

Dick RS, Steen EB (eds) (1991) The computer-based patient record. National Academy Press, Washington DC

Elmer-DeWitt P (1988) Fast and Smart. Time 131:54–58

Foresight Seminar on Pharmaceutical Research and Development (1989) Clinical trials in the 1990s: new methodologies for drug review. Washington DC March 22

Foresight Seminar on Pharmaceutical Research and Development (1991a) Evaluating cost effectiveness: future requirements for drug approval and reimbursement. Washington DC September 10

Foresight Seminar on Pharmaceutical Research and Development (1991b) Treatment protocols and outcome measures: future directions. Washington DC May 10

Foresight Seminar on Pharmaceutical Research and Development (1992) DUR: Beyond the Next Phase. Washington DC July 6

Gates W (1990) Interview. Washington Post, December 30: H1

Gilder G (1989) Microcosm. Simon and Schuster, New York

Gilder G (1991) Into the telecosm. Harvard Business Review, March-April: 150–161

High performance computing and communications act of 1991. H.R. 656, S. 272

Hooper L (1992) New mainframes fail to generate boom in revenue. Wall Street Journal, October 27: B3

Keller JJ (1992) No tongues too twisted for computer. Wall Street Journal, November 3: B4

Kluger J (1989) Private Screening. Discover, June: 32–34

Larson N (1992) Failure in the information age. MaxThink Journal. August: 1–6 (editorial)

Lipton HL, Bird JA (1991) Drug utilization review: state-of-the science and directions for outcomes research. Institute for Health Policy Studies, School of Medicine, University of California, San Francisco

Marketletter (1992) Marketletter Publications Limited 19: 26–27

Markoff J (1991) Xerox bobbled a brilliant computer vision in the 70s; it's trying again with 'ubiqutious computing'. New York Times, October 6:1

Mayo JS (1985) The evolution of information technologies. In: Guile BR (ed) Information technologies and social transformation. National Academy Press, Washington DC

McAleese R (ed) (1989) Hypertext: theory into practice. Blackwell, Oxford

MITI, Agency of Industrial Science and Technology (1987) A Vision of the Information Industry in the Year 2000. MITI Publication, June 19, pp 57–64

Moravec H (1988) Mind children. Harvard University Press, London

Naj AK (1991) Bacteria protein may help to miniaturize computers. Wall Street Journal, September 4:B5

Nelson TH (1987) Literary machines. The Author, San Antonio

Olson RL (1991) The upcoming transformation in health information systems. Address to the session on "Technology Developments for the 1990s" at the annual European Managers Meeting of IMS Corporation, Monte Carlo, January 1992

Olson RL, Bezold C (1990) Back to the future: revisiting the information millennium. Insight. Bell Communications Research Publication, pp 8–18

Olson RL, Jones MG, Bezold C (1992) 21st century learning and health care in the home: creating a national communications network. Institute for Alternative Futures, Alexandria, VA, and Consumer Interest Research Institute, Washington, DC

Omnibus Reconciliation Act (OBRA) (1990) Public Law 101–508, Section 4401: Reimbursement for Prescribed Drugs. November 5

Peck JC, Bezold C (1992) Health Care and AIDS. Ann Am Acad Poli Social Sci 522: 130–139

Peck JC, Rabin KH (1989) Regulating change: the regulation of foods, drugs, medical devices and cosmetics in the 1990s. Food and Drug Law Institute, Washington DC

Reindenberg MM (ed) (1991) Workshop on Drug Utilization Review, part 2 Clinical Pharmacol Ther 50 (5)

Scientific American (1991) Special Issue on Computers and Communication Networks, September (this is the best recent popular overview of major trends and developments)

Strauss W, Howe N (1991) Generations. William Morrow, New York

Sullivan LW (1992) New steps toward creating a nationwide electronic health information system. Remarks by the Secretary of Health and Human Services. Skokie, Illinois. October 19

Tank DW, Hopfield JJ (1987) Collective computation in neuronlike circuits. Sci Am 257:104–114

Toffler A (1980) The Third Wave. William Morrow, New York

Toffler A (1990) Power shift. Bantam, New York

Yoder SK (1992) Superfast chips inventively mix brain and brawn. Wall Street Journal, February 19: B1

Yonezawa A (1992) The real world computing program: MITI's next computer research initiative. Science 248: 581–582

Zachary GP (1992) Claim is made for improving display screens. Wall Street Journal, February 10: B1

# 2   2010: Culmination or Continuum?

Willis B. Goldbeck

Eighteen years from now, in the year 2010, we will have witnessed the greatest human revolution in recorded history. The drama ahead lies not in technology, but rather in the companion (some would say resulting) changes in human values and in social and political structures. Biotechnology, molecular nanotechnology, new drugs from space and undersea laboratories, the human genome project: these and many more conjure visions of disease eradication, an end to world hunger, sustainable development, and the proverbial "more life to our years as well as more years to our lives." Today, we know these developments in technology, and more as yet unimagined, are coming. We want to be filled with joy as well as expectation. But we have no idea today how we will cope with the results. Therein lies the ultimate challenge of the next 18 years. The management of innovation is far more complex than the process of innovation itself. We would be well advised to be wary if not deeply worried. This conclusion poses a significant challenge to the pharmaceutical industry, which has evidenced far more ability and willingness to deal effectively with the evolution of technology than with the more revolutionary aspects of social change.

## Scenarios

The scenarios prepared for this workshop present a rich and stimulating mosaic that virtually exhorts a pharmaceutical company to begin a process of constant self-examination. For introspection by an individual, company, or country to have value, it must take place within a constellation of information that challenges contemporary assumptions and forces new ways of analysis and communication upon people possessed of fine mind and strong will.

Scenarios are information tools that themselves grow in complexity and validity by repetitive use. Given the uncertainty of the timing and sequence of events in the next 18 years, it is hard to imagine a company emerging from this period as a real global success without a considerable investment in scenario-driven analysis and planning. This is especially true for institutions that are, by today's standards, already successful.

Serendipitous hot flashes of success are left to those that have yet to emerge. For the giants of today – already facing myriad social, economic, and political complexities that make the chemical compounds of pharma seem simple by comparison – there is no known substitute for the hard work of analysis and the never-ending cycles of vision development, strategic planning, and tactical implementation.

Combining scenarios with the generation and articulation of institutional vision will be one way leaders who come to their position by happenstance, history, or inheritance may actually retain – or attain – their lofty status during our transition into the next century.

Having clearly stated support for scenarios and vision (especially when integrated), I suggest that the primary trends and changes predicted for 2010 will take place regardless of which scenario option comes closest to reality. We must guard against the psychologically attractive trap that makes us think, and even desire, to have vision become synonymous with solution or prescription.

## Prediction and Trends

Working with scenarios can give insights of great value about when events may take place, the forces that may make those events more or less significant, and the opportunities an institution has to influence its own future. Scenarios can become misleading when they are given a reverence their authors would never invite. Analytical tools are to be used, even abused, but never revered. Seeking the "winning" scenario is no more than a simple way to avoid the intellectual challenge for which the scenarios were collectively designed. Predictions of future events and trends can be determined to be right or wrong at any given point in time. Scenarios are the screens through which predictions must pass and be measured.

With that in mind, the following health industry-related predictions are offered from the vantage point of the year 2010:

- Neither technology nor investment has been enough. More than 50 million people have died of AIDS and the end is not in sight despite the presence of a proven inoculation.
- Earth inhabitants are increasingly benefiting from space exploration, especially the recent space station-based laboratories. These are considered international property with joint ownership of all discoveries and joint investment from the public and private sectors of leading nations – an extension of the "common heritage" concept that evolved in the 1970s and 1980s regarding Antarctica. One result is that the pharmaceutical industry is now a partner with government, which is also the largest purchaser and distributor of pharma products.
- People are also suffering from the (inevitable) first disease(s) imported from space.
- Technology has answered the question about when life begins. Abortion is an issue only for populations too poor or unwilling to obtain any of the reliable long-term birth control regulators now available for men as well as women over the counter and through government programmes. One result is increased underground markets for healthy babies, fetal tissue, and baby organs for transplant. The United States and the European Community have led the effort for international conventions to prohibit commerce in human parts, but economic incentives and individual desperation are countervailing forces that are too strong.
- Human values are more severely challenged at the other end of the life cycle. Death on demand, self-initiated or by instructions, is easy to obtain and considered preferable to life prolonged at great expense and with low quality.
- The Triad is now the United States, Europe (including what were known as the newly independent states and about 30% of the former Commonwealth of Independent States), and China, including

eastern portions of the former Soviet Union. Japan acts as a regional military threat while, and perhaps because of, becoming less of a global economic power.

- The new generation of leaders has had to struggle to take full advantage of the new generation of opportunities. (Eighteen years is a long time in terms of innovation and social change, but all who would be leaders then are already here now; most have already finished college and selected the path they think will bring them success – as defined in 1990s' terms. The paucity of education, business, or public service programmes that provide training or even minimal analytical capacity to grapple with the future does not engender confidance that these individuals will be ready for the twenty-first century.) The global trend towards more women and younger men at the top brought increased pressure to implement a public vision of health products as public goods rather than the engines of corporate profits.

One risk of looking ahead 18 years is that we tend to think of this as a really long time when in fact it is dangerously short. More than 20 years have already passed since the end of the Vietnam War; life expectancy for millions is more than 18 years after age 65; and in the United States political system, 18 years is only three Senate terms.

On the other hand, the Single European Act – the critical event in the passage of the Treaty of Rome in 1957 to Maastricht in 1992 – was not signed until 1986, only 6 years ago.


## The View From 2010: Looking Back to See Ahead

At least five major trends over the past 18 years are reshaping health systems on both sides of the Atlantic, and revising our view of life itself.

- Professional data become public information
- From inspection to measurement, cost to value
- Aging, employment, and environmental immigration
- Triad or tribalism?
- Return of spirituality

## Professional Data Become Public Information

Advances in communications technology and its acceptance by the major public and private institutions responsible for health have been on a parallel track with the public's increased demand for control over the information that governs their health choices. Physicians are no longer gods in white but rather advisors of all colors. Every household has access to all the information now available to any health care professional and that includes the pharmaceutical industry and pharmacy itself. In turn, the pharmacy and the physician-led health office have all the information that enables matching a true patient profile with all the available interventions.

Individuals' use of medical care can be traced by codes for which confidentiality has been assured and social acceptance obtained. Benefits of public and private insurance are totally portable, at least throughout the United States and Europe.

Drugs are extremely popular and respected, but all must be shown to have value, measured in some balance of health, pleasure, and cost. The process of gaining public acceptance of legal drugs for the purpose of pleasure rather than cure or prevention has been one of the more dramatic and contentious social transformations, and the single most profitable for the drug industry.

The health systems of Europe and the United States have moved closer to a single model, with the social equity and income distribution commitments of Europe being balanced by successful U.S. cost control and cost distribution mechanisms.

European countries now spend on average 12% of their gross national or domestic products on health, while spending in the United States stabilized at 16% in 1999. Nevertheless, the public satisfaction with health care delivery – the feeling of a return on investment and thus political support – has grown significantly since the low point of 1995.

The role of nurses, home health aides, and new classes of health helpers has expanded as the role of physicians became increasingly restricted to technology management, research, and diagnostic procedures. At the same time, physicians are making house calls again now that there is a telematics connection between every physician's pocket telephone and the world's medical information systems.

### From Inspection to Measurement, Cost to Value

The power of the information revolution also fuels the desire by consumers and health professionals alike to shift from systems of inspection
to a new spirit of public accountability focused on measured results. In
the case of pharmaceuticals, the era of recording adverse drug reactions
has been replaced by automatic measurement of all drug use, and by
public disclosure of the outcomes. Data are voice-entered, reducing
physician opposition to the increased administrative demands. Every
hospital and long-term-care bed is connected to distributed fiber optic
computing networks with CD-ROM video, image, and voice capacity
(hypermedia). The multilingual nature of this technology leads directly
to increased patient satisfaction and expands employment opportunities
among immigrant groups. This massive new data access led to the first
serious post-market surveillance of drug experience.

Global access to standardized information through open systems
architecture (largely ISDN and increased broadband) resulted in the
globalization of the health care industry. Primary regulatory mechanisms are the same in all First World countries and increasingly in the
second tier. "Special cases" and some national industry subsidies linger,
but they are clear exceptions and often relate to shared objectives such
as the European Community's multi-billion ECU fund to assist infrastructure development in the "poorest" member nations. This programme, a continuation of efforts in the 1980s and 1990s to improve
development in Greece, Ireland, Portugal, and Spain, is now applied
primarily to countries of the former eastern Europe and represents a
blending of traditional foreign aid with targeted industrial development
assistance. Health care companies, especially those that combine individual care products and services with community environmental clea-
nup and protection products and services, are a favourite of this investment strategy.

The "winners" in the pharma and health products industries are those
that invested in new markets rather than increasing their competitive
position in existing ones – those that understood that their product and
service was health (not the pills and potions, which were only the
vehicles), thus removing historical loyalty to or rejection of generics,
research, direct advertising, or other artefacts of mid-nineteenth century
values.

Value, particularly for personal health products and services, will increasingly be measured in explicit economic terms as centralized payment systems that can afford and manage the full capacity of existing comparative data systems become the primary purchasers. Value is also measured by the public's feeling of improvements in quality of life. How to make such measurements on a publicly comparative basis was a topic of major social and economic research in the late 1990s. Health care industry leaders are those who have been able to correctly predict shifts in social values and thus gear their products and services to coincide with these measures, as well as being able to prove that their products passed the economic value tests of the day. Formularies are much more restrictive than they were in the boom 1980s. Health status improves as a result of a combination of monitored usage and reduced financial barriers to a more tightly controlled "cabinet" of products of proven quality.

## Aging, Employment, and Environmental Immigration

In the United States, Japan, and Europe, the aging of the population combined with below-replacement-level rates of birth (for all but Ireland) meant there were both too few workers to generate the income to pay for social programmes and not enough workers of the right skills to take advantage of the health-related technology that was developed during the past 18 years.

These countries (the old Triad) adopted policies of extracting labour from the same developing countries from which the extraction of natural resources fueled the industrial revolution. The early twenty-first century parallel to the former dependence of First World countries on Third World oil is dependence on Third World peoples for labour, but no longer only for "cheap" or "undesirable" tasks. Policies that were ostensibly to improve the Third World in fact became systematic "brain drain" programmes that further delayed movements of economic independence in Africa, Asia, Latin America, and the Middle East. The results were small temporary benefits and large long-term problems as payments for greatly increased military operations throughout the world far exceeded the value of the skills exploited. Ironically, following historical patterns, medical technology was a direct beneficiary of continued conflict.

Compounding these problems were the pressures of spasmodic mass migration due to environmental disasters. More than a decade of talking did little to prevent Chernobyl II and even more widespread disasters from reactors in Bulgaria and Romania. The inextricable links between energy, employment, and health policies became increasingly apparent.

Millions of refugees fleeing environmental or human-caused disasters altered the history of migration, straining the fibers of tolerance and creating a new demand for chemical products to replace many natural foods and even the life-giving properties of potable water.

Advances in transportation and telemedicine have had the positive effect of extending to the poorest regions the latest preventive and curative services from the most advanced centres and staff in London, Paris, or New York. Payment for such services, on an internationally agreed fee schedule, is administered through the United Nations and has proved to be less expensive than the large-scale relief efforts of the 1990s. Without it having been made explicit, the First World found such systems of global equalization to be a reasonable down payment on its investment in Third World labour and a more predictable resource allocation than traditional foreign aid programmes were.

### Triad or Tribalism?

The concept of the Triad is a bit like the men's clubs of the early twentieth century: comfort provided by common purpose masking the real differences among members. The historical connections between Western Europe and the United States were easy to understand. Inclusion of Japan would more properly be viewed as an attempt by the former two to keep a check on their World War II enemy, which threatened to do far more lasting damage with economic power than it had ever achieved with military fanaticism. This view gained credibility in 2004 when Japan was replaced by China. In effect, a market of sudden wealth (Japan) was being replaced by a much larger market of people (China). The fact that China was the world's largest, if not most sophisticated, military power and had growing economic clout through the extension of Hong Kong's success inland contributed to the apparent reasonableness of their new status.

Unfortunately, the Triad, regardless of change in membership, did not represent the significant political trend of the era. The flash points of Yugoslavia became more rule than exception as the major powers and their international institutions displayed inherent inabilities to prevent or halt what were in effect tribal conflicts. Long thought to be limited to the less developed regions (a concept that could only have its origins among those who entitled themselves "more" developed), ethnic and religious conflicts raced across the face of Europe, the Indian continent, Asia, Africa, and the Middle East. Latin America was the shining exception, as its common Catholic heritage and strengthened ties with the United States proved mutually supportive.

From a health care perspective, the altered Triad increased access to the Chinese millions and unleashed a major expansion of competing pharma companies based on product lines of "eastern" medicines and therapies.

Whatever positive impact resulted from the Triad was more than offset by the negative consequences of tribalism. Conflicts at the turn of the century involved displacement of millions and caused unprecedented pressure on the health and social welfare systems of Western nations. Mass arrivals of peoples with different nutritional traditions, new physical and spiritual needs, and a lack of economic independence threatened to turn all Western health facilities into triage units resembling those made famous by the old American TV show M*A*S*H. The heated discussions about rationing of care that had characterized the health care reform movement of the 1990s seemed distant and irrelevant as the demands for medical and health services totally surpassed the wealth of any nation to respond favourably. Formal systems of rationing were the only alternative to riots on health care access, and the manner in which this issue was managed became a political survival test that many a Western leader failed.

## Return of Spirituality

Early humans (including such later-day populations as the American Indian) understood that they were one manifestation of nature. Humans could not be healthy if nature was not also. Concepts of sharing, universality, spirituality, mutuality, and the nexus of physical and emotional health all come from a basic, intuitive understanding of the total and permanent integration of humanity with nature.

Humans' institutions and our modern icons have emphasized the separation of humanity from nature, or, worse, the superiority of human beings over nature. The ways in which people today desire and seek health, select life-styles, set priorities, respect the environment, and allocate effort and resources are all reflections of values.

The articulation of our health desires and demands represents the changing literature of the evolution of values. In the 1980s and 1990s, language began to reflect the growing awareness that medicine and technology represented only a small fraction of the total influences on human health. Life-styles, personal behaviour, the interplay of humans and their institutions of work and play, of habitat and education, sustainable development rather than environmental extraction and exploitation, self-esteem – these and many others were attempts to bring balance to a world in which ill health was defined by violence, accidents, environmental degradation, crowding, hunger, homelessness, AIDS, smoking, alcohol, drugs, and sedentary living.

The technology that humans so idolized could not solve the problems they had also invented. Child immunization is a near-perfect technology, but only when accessible to all; prenatal care works, but not if avoided; billions are spent treating cancer and cardiovascular diseases we could simply decide not to get. (See Appendix for guidance on reading and other materials on a new public health philosophy.)

Humans entered the twenty-first century with the technological accomplishments of the past serving largely to display the weaknesses of the present. Technology was not the problem.

At the turn of the century, fueled by the threats and promises of past religious leaders, spirituality lost ground to those who sought and perhaps truly believed that one brand of faith was, could, or should be superior. In the ensuing decade the fallacy of this approach became ever more clear and the year 2010 will long be known as the watershed when the concept of true spirituality, the elusive integration of mind and body, transcended the individual and became inculcated in a time of societal renewal.

## Conclusion

A song popular in the United States in the 1950s said, "the future is not ours to see . . . whatever will be will be . . .". Today, in 1992, our vision is a lot clearer and the view is one filled with delight and daring as well as potential demons. Increasingly, we exercise control over our future, or at least appear to do so until the next blast of nature reminds us how small we really are and how important that comprehensive spirituality must be.

In health, we really do have the power: our personal and collective decisions about life-style remain the largest determinant of our future. Technology is a fabulous asset not only to the correction or removal of a specific problem but also for the expansion of the entire spectrum of human knowledge from which further strides in progress and prevention will surely come.

Technology also holds the promise of contributing to increased equity throughout the world, a goal that is often relegated to the dreamers but without which none of us will ever be free to fully enjoy the richness of our opportunity here on spaceship earth.

## Appendix

The most important health documents of the late twentieth century provide some insight to those in search for a new (some would argue renewed) public health philosophy and commitment.

Foremost is the "bible" of the World Health Organization (WHO), *Health for All*. Especially as expressed in the work of the WHO European Region, there has never been a better articulation of a grand vision, complete with strategy, tactics, and measurable targets for implementation of an integrated public health policy, programme, and practice involving literally all aspects of human society.

The United States made a major contribution with the preparations of *Healthy People 2000*, a detailed and dynamic guide to the attainment of significantly improved health for the next century.

*The European Charter for Health and the Environment*, a more modest volume than the two above, was created by the European Regional Office of WHO in collaboration with the European Community.

It is the most specific prescription for the integration of health and environmental policy that the political process has accomplished.

In the *New Treaty on European Unity*, the European Community gave its political institutions a new Public Health Authority – rich in purpose, mercifully brief, and clear of spirit.

"The Community shall contribute towards ensuring a high level of human health protection by encouraging cooperation between the member states and, if necessary, lending support to their action".

"Community action shall be directed towards the prevention of diseases, in particular the major health scourges, including drug dependence, by promoting research into their causes and their transmission, as well as health information and education".

"Health protection demands shall form a constituent part of the Community's other policies".

"Member states shall, in liaison with the Commission, co-ordinate among themselves their policies and programmes in the areas (above)".

"The Commission may, in close contact with the member states, take any useful initiative to promote such co-ordination".

"The Community and member states shall foster co-operation with third countries and the competent international organizations in the sphere of public health."

The health industry of today would be well served to notice that the directions for tomorrow do not include one word about technology or medical care.

Another publication well worth reading is Michael Murphy's *The Future of the Body: Explorations into the Future Evolution of Human Nature* (J.P. Tarcher, 1992).

Finally, there is a remarkable 13-volume video series by Joseph Campbell, *Transformation of Myth Through Time*. No finer declaration of humanity's inherent unity with nature has been presented.

# 3 The Future of Pharmaceutical Therapy and Regulation

Louis Lasagna

## The Physicians of Tomorrow

Physicians will continue to be dominant in decisions about drug prescribing, but clinical pharmacists employed by hospitals and health maintenance organizations will exert power in formulary decisions and in drug purchasing negotiations. Marketing must take this into account.

The training of physicians will move in two opposite directions – the production of "generalists" (family physicians, internists, and pediatricians) to meet the needs and preferences of patients who do not want to be treated by "committees," and the production of super-specialists to handle complex diagnostic and therapeutic maneuvers that cannot be properly managed by physicians lacking the requisite training and experience. This situation already obtains to a significant degree, but the differences will be magnified as the years go by. Nevertheless, generalists will continue to prescribe most types of drugs.

This situation is analogous to what is happening in all of science and industry: the need for detailed, focused expertise combined with the need to integrate new knowledge and techniques into an effective gestalt.

## Changes in Public Attitudes

The public will change in important ways. Industrial countries will undergo an acceleration of the "graying" process, with higher percentages of elderly citizens who will require some sort of health care but who will be least able to pay for it, either with taxes or out-of-pocket expenditures. (I will return to this issue later.)

Activists will become more powerful, following the lead (and successes) of the AIDS lobby and the animal rights movement. Patient advocates will press industry, regulatory agencies, and government-supported researchers to explain and justify the slow pace of development of needed new remedies, especially for life-threatening illnesses, while the animal rights groups will seek to eliminate all animal research.

Younger and better educated members of society will not be content to be passive recipients of medical care. They will seek to be partners with physicians in making diagnostic and therapeutic choices. To do this efficiently, they will want more and better information about both disease and treatment. Generations comfortable with computers will be ripe for educational material especially produced for interactive computer systems. There will be pressure for more "direct-to-consumer" advertisements and rejection of the right of paternalistic government censors to restrict the access of citizens to information that may improve the quality of their choices.

## Unmet Needs

Gaps in our medical armamentarium will require research to be targeted either on improving treatments already available or on providing new medicines for diseases where no worthwhile remedies exist. Preferably, these new discoveries will be "blockbuster" advances of major impact, but modest gains will still be more probable and will not be unappreciated. A new, palatable liquid medication or chewable tablet for children may seem like a trivial scientific accomplishment, but it may confer dramatic benefits, and it constitutes real progress.

Cures will be the goal, but symptomatic improvement will be the rule. Elimination of disease will occur only with the development of effective vaccines distributed on a global basis. Cancer, degenerative diseases, and AIDS will all increase in frequency.

There will be a demand for ways to "fine-tune" treatment, identifying in advance, rather than by trial and error, which available treatment is best for a specific patient. This will require changes both in protocol design and in retrospective analysis of data from clinical trials. A. Bradford Hill, in a lecture given a quarter of a century ago, complained of the inability of controlled trials to tell physicians what they wanted to know about a drug: how to use it optimally in individual patients, not groups of patients.

Certain patient–physician groups will champion the cause of "melioristic" pharmacology, the goal of which will be not the remedy of somatic or mental derangements but rather the achievement of a "supernormal" state of health, with health being defined not as just the absence of disease but as the maximum fulfillment of mental and physical potential.

## Opportunities for New Products

Leads for new remedies will arise from many quarters. The human genome project will identify genetic loci for most diseases and provide clues for new therapeutic approaches, including gene therapy. Progress here will be slow, however. (Recall that it is now several decades since the genetic basis of sickle cell anemia was described in detail, without any effective therapy having resulted to date.) Gene sequencing will ultimately provide important advances, but not in the near future.

Biotechnology will continue to grow in importance, as biologically important proteins are manufactured and incorporated into medical progress. The pace of success will be slower than in the pre-1992 period because searching, for instance, for cures for cancer or for immunomodulators provides a greater challenge than was the case for human insulin, human growth hormone, or erythropoietin.

Molecular genetics and antisense compounds will be even more difficult to apply practically because of our inability to predict the results of such approaches. Endogenous proteins and growth factors will receive attention because they obviously play a role in the body's economy, and therefore modulation of such materials is likely to cause important perturbations, sometimes desirable and other times not.

X-ray crystallography, magnetic resonance imaging, and new visual graphic techniques, combined with computer analysis, will provide new ways to predict utility and toxicity. Rational drug design will take precedence over empiric "screening," but will not replace the latter because the database for such rational design and our ability to predict pharmacokinetic functions and adverse reactions remains limited.

New drug delivery systems will not only be a source of market exclusivity, they will improve bioavailability and compliance with prescribing directions.

To increase the likelihood of "breakthrough" drugs, scientists in industry, academia, and government laboratories will increasingly cooperate. Research and development agreements will grow in number for situations where drugs were developed mainly (or exclusively) by federal or private foundation funds.

## Pressures on the Pharmaceutical Industry

A variety of pressures on industry will increase. Cost analyses will be routinely demanded to help decide whether registration or reimbursement by third-party payors is deserved. Simple cost analysis is easy but only applicable where different treatments give identical clinical outcomes.

Cost-effectiveness analysis will be needed where treatments differ in the extent to which they meet one unambiguous objective (such as prolongation of life). Cost-utility analysis, while quite complex, will be preferred where impacts on the quality of life are important or where there are trade-offs (between, for example, length and quality of life). Cost-benefit analysis, while appropriate where both costs and benefits are quantifiable in monetary terms alone, will often not be applicable because so much of health care involves both monetary and nonmonetary costs and benefits.

Reimbursement will be readily granted for major breakthroughs or for drugs specifically effective for a definable target subpopulation.

International harmonization will decrease, but not eliminate, intercountry differences with regard to drug registration, and industry will have to battle the tendency for regulatory requirements to become excessive and inflexible. There will be a centralized clearinghouse to facilitate drug registration in Europe, but no "Super Food and Drug Administration." Nations will retain the right to individualize drug approval, drug rejection, removal of drugs from the market, and the status of "traditional" remedies. Japan and the United States will continue to depend on their own regulatory agencies. "Local" or "national" pharmaceutical firms will receive favored treatment by government regulators and pricing authorities in both Europe and Japan.

Failure to develop enough new drugs, and especially the always rare blockbusters, will force mergers or facilitate takeovers. Some firms will cease all significant research and development (R&D) activity and try to exist on old products or licensed ones. Many small biotech firms will fail, as will some small generic houses. The world economy will not return to earlier expansive levels, although China and some developing countries will improve their economic status and provide new markets for products from industrial countries. The business environment will remain unstable.

Drug pricing will continue to be the Achilles' heel of the pharmaceutical industry. Companies will have to defend their pricing policies and explain variations in price from country to country. Generic and even therapeutic substitution will be encouraged by governments in attempts to contain health care costs and to get around patent exclusivity. Individual countries will differ in their preferences for controlling drug prices, volume of drugs used, or drug profits. Parallel imports will decrease.

There will be conflict between politicians and voters who support a vigorous and innovative drug industry and those who prefer a mildly profitable industry that becomes in essence a public utility, providing at low prices the fruits of past research but not of the future. The United States, formerly the last bastion of free drug pricing, will move towards federal price control, at least for patients covered by government programs. Special discounts will be demanded for all such programs. Local communities and hospitals will all institute drug utilization review programs.

All nations will set caps on the percentage of gross domestic product they wish to spend on health care. This will entail a draconian elimination of all drug expenses deemed unjustifiable or excessively expensive. Because the ability to trim "fat" out of the health care budget is limited but the ability of science to come up with new diagnostic tests, drugs, surgical procedures, prostheses, organ transplants, and so on is not, rationing of health care is inevitable.

Complaints about rationing will lead to some increased taxes and supplementary voluntary health insurance plans or out-of-pocket purchases. Some national health insurance schemes will go bankrupt, or will avoid bankruptcy only by substantially increasing copayments and deductibles. Younger taxpayers will be resentful of the need to pay for services for elderly patients who pay no taxes. It is even possible to imagine pressures to shorten the lives of oldsters in nursing homes who are living lives devoid of either personal satisfaction or social utility.

Especially troubling will be the problem of paying for important therapeutic breakthroughs (such as a cure for muscular dystrophy) if such breakthroughs are extremely expensive to supply and deliver. Failure to pay for such advances will help the national health care budget but at an enormous price in terms of social guilt and the de-meaning of societal values.

## Decreasing Health Care Costs

Although drugs are an easy target for federal cost containment bureau-crats, other targets exist. More attempts will be made to give home health care so as to decrease the use of expensive hospital or nursing home beds. Prevention of disease by exercise, nutrition, and screening programs will be encouraged. In Japan, physicians will increasingly give way to pharmacists as dispensers of medicines.

With regard to drug-related harm, liability schemes similar to those in place for some years in, for example, Sweden and Finland will be adopted by most countries. Punitive damages will be outlawed where state-of-the-art defense is applicable.

## Decreasing R&D Costs in Industry

Realization of the importance of improving the efficiency of drug devel-opment will lead to some changes. Regulatory agencies will be asked to set forth, in explicit terms, the calculus of risk and benefit used for new drug approval. Prompt and equitable appeal mechanisms will be put in place to deal with disagreements between the regulators and the regu-lated.

More modest data requirements will be combined with additional postapproval research to provide needed information that is considered not significant enough to delay registration. Improved pharmacoepidemiologic techniques will be devised, including data recording on new drugs (and perhaps old) via computer networks in doctors' offices.

The processing of new drug data both before and after submission for regulatory approval will be facilitated by the use of computer-assisted techniques. New drug applications will be scrutinized by professional extragovernmental firms (approved by the local regulatory agency) with access to the requisite statistical, clinical, and toxicologic skills to speed reviews. New drug applications will be of sufficiently high quality and completeness that they do not delay the approval process by requiring new studies or analyses.

## The Need for Diversification

To increase the chances for survival, pharmaceutical firms will diversify their product lines to include generic drugs (versions of their own formerly patented chemicals or versions of other companies' off-patent drugs), over-the-counter remedies, "nutriceutical" products (such as fat substitutes), miniaturized portable health records, diagnostic tests and machines, imaging technology, and computer programs for lay or physician users to improve individual health care and drug prescribing.

While innovative firms have in the past fought generic competition by appealing to physician prescriber loyalty, in the future specific countries will demand generic substitution as a cost-saving measure, in which case the innovative companies will decide to compete with non-innovative multidrug sources by offering comparable prices but using time-tested performance and physician loyalty as positive selling points.

## The Opening Up of Foreign Markets

Japanese and European drug companies that are not now significantly multinational in scope will attempt to invade foreign markets to make up for decreasing profits in their home markets. Japan will allow foreign firms increased access to the Japanese market in return for absence of interference with Japanese pharmaceutical presence in the United States and Europe.

## Government Drug Development

If public sector pressures for treatment of "orphan diseases" cannot be resisted politically, governments will play an initiating and continuing role in the development of "orphan drugs" for rare diseases. The political skill of patient advocacy groups will determine how much (if any) R&D efforts will be devoted to a search for remedies for such diseases.

# 4 The Pharmaceutical Industry in 2010

Barrie G. James

The environment of the pharmaceutical industry has been relatively stable since the late 1950s. The industry adopted a producer orientation to serve a global market characterized by low sensitivity to price, a relatively large gap between the knowledge of manufacturers and customers, and a very tenuous linkage between cost awareness and cost containment. This enabled companies to follow long-run policies of selling what they could find and make at premium prices. There was little fear of a real competitive challenge, as competition was based not on price but on the ability to introduce a steady stream of patent-protected new products into a steadily growing market.

This producer orientation began to crumble in the late 1980s and early 1990s as the environment began to change. From now on success for pharmaceutical companies will not be linked almost exclusively to their ability to find and develop new products but instead to their ability to respond to the new forces driving change.

This chapter outlines those key forces, profiles three fundamental industry structural trends, and concludes with a "best guess" picture of the pharmaceutical industry in 2010.

## Driving Forces of Change

The pharmaceutical industry is facing a range of powerful forces that are reshaping its environment.

**Health Care Delivery**

In almost all countries the ability of public and private health care systems to meet the continuous demand for all forms of health care has reached a point where medical capabilities outstrip the means to pay. This crisis in health care costs is being driven by a number of issues:

- Demographic change, with low birth rates and improvements in health care, is extending the human life cycle and the demand for resources in industrial countries. Growing economic prosperity in newly industrializing nations is increasing demand, while in the Third World demand is linked to population but decoupled from the ability to pay.
- The ease of access, particularly in public-sector systems, has led to overconsumption of scarce resources.
- As established diseases are brought under control, diseases more difficult and expensive to diagnose and treat are emerging.
- The growing incidence of noncommunicable life-style diseases, which can be prevented through informed choice and early detection, are driving up treatment costs.
- The provision of health care has become a major industry attracting high salaries, costly equipment, and inflexible infrastructures.

Since the late 1950s, most public health care systems have imposed and then accelerated their controls over price, volume, and promotion and have introduced deregulation to contain health care costs. With poor public recognition and no political support, the pharmaceutical industry has borne a disproportionate share of these escalating supply side controls.

The political realization from the early 1980s that health care expenditures were out of control and that demographic and life-style patterns for the 1990s indicated inevitable increases in consumption in pharmaceutical products prompted a new set of practices to manage demand. Initiatives were introduced that promoted cost awareness to decision

**Fig. 1.** Cost containment linkage: influencing market size and growth, pricing, margins and competition (from James 1992)

| Approach | Supply side | Demand side | Impact on manufacturers |
|---|---|---|---|
| Focus | Policies | Practices | |
| Targets and measures | Cost reduction | Cost awareness | |
| | Companies:<br>Profit control (UK)<br>Physician access (Sweden)<br>Compulsory licences (Canada)<br>Cost plus pricing (Spain)<br>Reimbursement (Italy)<br>Price comparisons (France)<br>• Generic substitution (various)<br>• Formularies (USA)<br>• Biennial price reductions (Japan)<br>• Parallel imports (EC)<br>• Promotional spend tax (UK)<br>• Price/volume controls (France)<br>• Group buying (USA)<br>• Reference pricing (Germany)<br>• Therapeutic substitution (Germany)<br>• Registration fees (UK)<br>• Pharmacoeconomics (Australia) | Physicians:<br>Prescriber monitoring (UK)<br>• Positive lists (Spain)<br>• Negative lists (UK)<br>• Efficiency incentives (UK)<br>• Penalties for ineffiency (Germany)<br><br>Patients<br>Prescribing changes (UK)<br>No. items per script (UK)<br>• Increasing co-payment (Italy)<br>• Restricting access (Spain)<br>• Delisting products (France)<br><br>Pharmacies<br>• Excess profil repayments (UK)<br>• Incentives for substitution (Canada)<br>• Pharmacy prescribing (USA)<br><br>Combination:<br>• Rx to OTC switch (Denmark) | → <br>• Low growth market<br>• Segment declines<br>• Intensified |
| | (• Instituted from 1980s) | | |

Source: Pharma Strategy in "Pharmaceuticals: The New Marketing", The Economist Intelligence Unit, Special Report, R 201, 1992

making physicians, to patient users, and to pharmacy and wholesaler suppliers.

During the early 1990s it was recognized that by simultaneously pressuring the supply side with cost reduction policies and the demand side with a range of cost awareness practices, public and private health care insurers could contain costs (Fig. 1). However, this linkage has a much more profound implication for the pharmaceutical industry. It allows insurers to influence prices, volume, profits, market share, and the level of competition in the market place.

Essentially, the health care delivery cost crisis is a direct result of the long-run reluctance of governments to make sensible but politically unpopular decisions on the allocation of scarce resources. Since it is unlikely that governments will take the political risk or underwrite the costs of the massive realignments necessary to produce more affordable health care, both users and suppliers will be faced with continuous pressures on demand and supply. The way that insurers manage their new-found ability to simultaneously influence the supply and demand processes in the pharmaceutical market will have a powerful effect on the development of the pharmaceutical industry and the fortunes of individual companies.

## Customers

Fundamental changes under way in the structure of the pharmaceutical industry's customer base are shifting power away from traditional customers to a wide range of new groups. Driving this realignment are the twin forces of increasing customer knowledge in a value-for-money environment and the fusion of the supply chain.

-   Industry customers across the board have become increasingly knowledgeable about pharmaceutical products and their expectations have increased. Coupled with a greater emphasis on value-for-money decision making, this has resulted in the growing usage of cost and performance criteria in prescribing and purchasing decisions. Expanding customer knowledge is clashing with pharmaceutical companies as customers become unwilling to pay premiums for what they perceive are increasingly standardized products.

- Progressive changes in the economics and politics of health care and consumerism are fusing together the traditionally discrete links – user, prescriber, insurer, wholesaler, pharmacist, and regulator – in the pharmaceutical supply chain.

These two changes collectively present the pharmaceutical industry with a radically new environment in terms of what, how, and to whom they communicate and supply.

In the industrial world, companies are facing a plethora of customer groups, each with its own set of complex agendas: For the first time patients have become a new target audience, gaining choice at the point of prescribing and of dispensing. In many countries the decision-making power of the physician is eroding as prescribing is channeled by insurers into narrower cost-effective therapeutic product selections. Insurers are beginning to use their volume of purchases to extract significant price concessions for new products and adopt therapeutic substitution to optimize their funds. Wholesalers and pharmacies are consolidating and vertically integrating to improve their competitive position and protect their margins. Regulators are expanding their sphere of operations beyond product approvals by adopting economic criteria designed to improve the cost-effectiveness of drug therapy.

The pharmaceutical market in industrial countries is no longer a place but a network of interests. These powerful interlinked customer groups have the ability to leverage demand, supply, and distribution to suit their own economic agendas – at the expense of pharmaceutical companies.

**Technology**

Competition in the pharmaceutical industry has been built almost exclusively around the ability to find, fund, develop, and market new products by either developing new or modifying existing chemical structures. While the store of new technology continues to grow, offering the possibility of maintaining this competitive policy, the pharmaceutical industry faces two major problems:

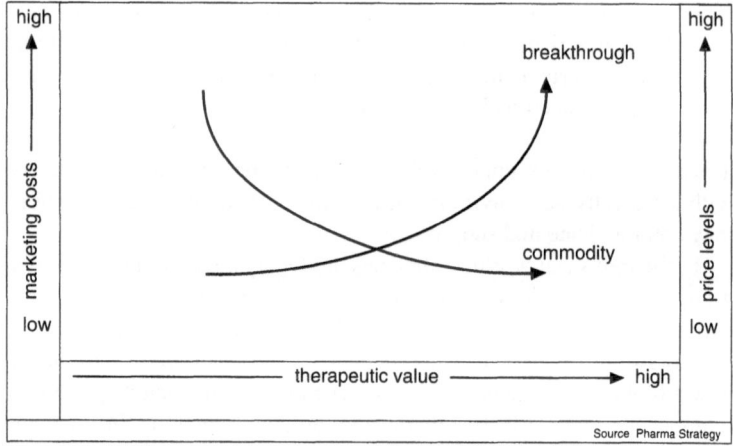

Source Pharma Strategy

**Fig. 2.** Price and cost implications of therapeutic value are forcing companies to use marketing to focus innovation (from James 1992)

1. Moving up the technology evolution curve is incurring exponential cost increases. Fewer companies can fund or accept the risk of developing cutting-edge technology for new therapies for long-term chronic diseases, because costs go up in multiples as a product moves from research through development to marketing.
2. Customers now have the ability to make rational selection decisions based on their perceptions of cost-effectiveness, and they are increasingly refusing to pay premiums for products they do not believe offer value-for-money.

Pharmaceutical companies are being squeezed by rising new product costs and the growing reluctance of customers to pay the increased costs for new products (Fig. 2). Customers are no longer buying new technology in the form of new products; instead, they are buying solutions to problems that meet their therapeutic value and economic expectations. The way pharmaceutical companies manage the trade-off between customer value (price) and their cost will be a critical success factor as the market dictates a shift from an industry-wide policy of "selling what you can make" to "making what you can sell."

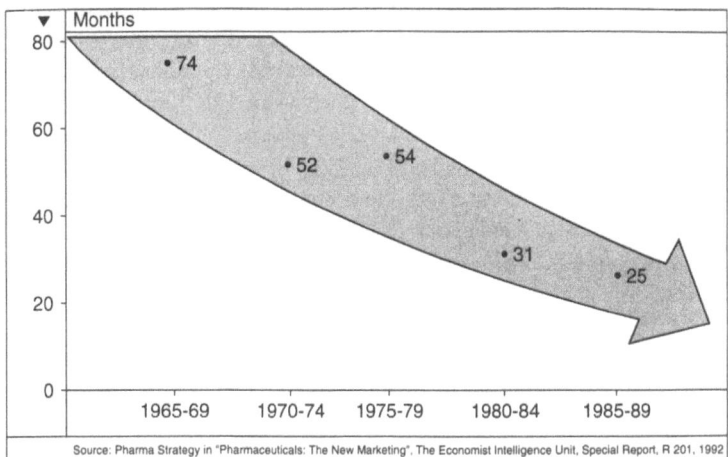

**Fig. 3.** Time elapsed between pioneer product launches and the first follow-on market entry, 1965–1989 (UK) (from James 1992)

## Competition

The basis of competition is changing radically in the pharmaceutical industry, driven by a number of converging trends:

- Despite increasing product complexity, the gap between innovator and follower has shrunk between the 1960s and the 1990s by two thirds (Fig. 3). Technology now matures more quickly, enabling competitors to duplicate innovative breakthroughs much faster with a follow-up product, which significantly reduces the exclusivity of innovators and the premiums they are able to charge.
- The growing chemical and clinical similarity of many new products and the bunching of introductions is helping reduce customers' perceptions of differences between products.
- Fewer companies can provide the internal funding for developing and marketing new products, with industry costs of $200 million for a major new product and $200 million for introducing a new product in the eight key markets that account for 70% of global pharmaceutical consumption.

- The growth of alternative therapies spurred by consumer dissatis-faction with traditional drug therapy, the increasing integration of prevention, diagnosis, and treatment, and the rise of prescription to over-the-counter (OTC) switches designed to place more of the fin-ancial burden on patients are all beginning to challenge the concept of a pure prescription market.
- The key world markets are continuing their marginal growth in prescriptions and unit volume; success is no longer a question of participating in a growing market where there is a place for all but of taking business away from other companies.

The simple model of pharmaceutical industry competition anchored in the ability to develop a stream of patent-protected new products is beginning to degrade in the face of a decline in exclusivity, a reduction in differentiation, increasing consumer sophistication, rising operating costs, the blurring of the market, and sharply increased levels of compe-tition. As the traditional competitive model becomes obsolete, success will be heavily geared to the critical decisions that pharmaceutical companies make on how, where, and with whom they wish to compete.

**Market Structure**

The pharmaceutical market in the industrial world is beginning to re-structure along the lines of the ability and willingness of customers to pay for drug therapy. Increasing cost containment linked to customer knowledge are driving the market into a number of new demand seg-ments determined by customers' perceptions of value-for-money (Fig. 4).

Market restructuring is creating a number of new realities:

- There are no guarantees that the market values all new technology. The traditional approach to developing new products – where "new" and "technology" conferred "better" and created the sales push – is fading. The dominant factor in the production process, in an era of cost containment and sophisticated customers, is price.
- The growth in parity products and customer knowledge is driving price erosion for newly introduced products.

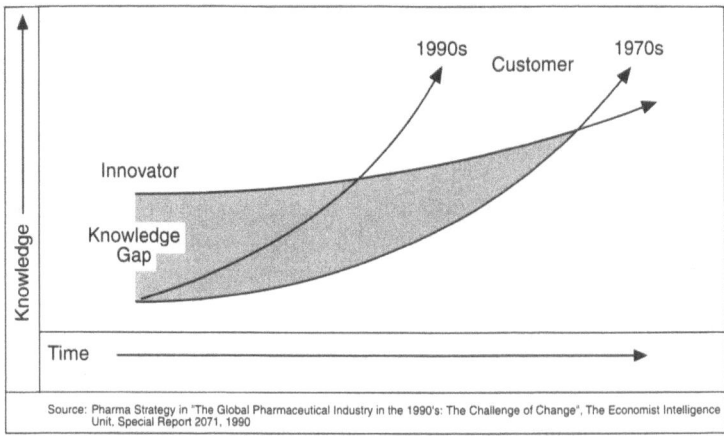

**Fig. 4.** Perceptions of therapeutic value. Increasing customer knowledge will focus greater attention in purchasing and prescribing on perceptions of therapeutic value (from James 1990)

– Deregulation has created the means to supply the price-sensitive segment of the market and growing demand has created a substantial generic business that has siphoned off the industry's traditional source of long-run profits.

The restructuring of the demand patterns holds major implications for the type of new product selected for development, the development process itself, and research, development, and manufacturing costs.

## Alternative Structural Trends

These key forces driving change have many implications for the future structure of the pharmaceutical industry. Alternative structural trends based on three specific models – consolidation, integration, and devolution – are discussed in this section.

## Consolidation

Unlike any other industry, the pharmaceutical business is characterized by a vast number of companies – some 7000 world-wide – with the largest ones having a market share of around 5% of the global pharmaceutical market.

Although sales are fragmented, innovation is concentrated: some 50 companies, all located in the industrial world, account for 70% of all industry innovation. These same companies are directly responsible for about 50% of global sales and indirectly, with licensing and comarketing arrangements, for a further 10% of sales.

Industry consolidation is favored by a number of factors:

*Access to technology:* A strong pipeline of products with a high level of clinical significance are becoming essential to secure prices high enough to pay for rising costs of innovation. The key issue is access to enough new ideas and enough cash to convert research concepts into high value-added new products. In the past, most companies could find and fund new products; now, however, higher costs combined with increasingly more complex technology and the demands of more sophisticated customers are driving an increase in innovation costs.

*Access to markets:* Molecules are born globally but largely marketed regionally or multinationally. The cost of innovation and rapid follow-on competition are forcing the development of global registration and marketing networks to introduce and commercialize new products rapidly and to achieve greater volume for acceptable returns on investment and risk.

*Competition:* More aggressive competition, rapid follow-on products, and high marketing costs with large sales forces are visible examples of the increase in style and type of competition. The two main sectors of consolidation that are emerging are mega-mergers (designed to obtain global leverage by expanding competitive mass in innovation, marketing, cash, and skills) and selective acquisitions aimed at strengthening a company's geographic, product, or technology portfolio.

More than at any other time in the industry's history, size is becoming a critical issue in finding and funding new technology and marketing new products on a global scale. In addition, the industry's four mega-mergers – Bristol Myers-Squibb, SmithKline-Beecham, Rhone Pou-lenc-Rorer, and Marion-Merrell Dow – have changed the ground rules. These new entities have created a larger critical mass in innovation, marketing, cash, and talent, and have also eliminated some of the op-tions of the other players. Already in France a number of medium-sized national companies have either merged with larger French companies or have sold out to multinationals from other countries.

Consolidation would move the pharmaceutical industry much closer to other industry models such as aerospace, automobiles, and consumer electronics, in which competitive mass is critical to leveraging the market in breadth globally and in depth nationally. Typically, a very small number of very large companies dominate such industries, with niche companies supplying specific customer needs and meeting geo-graphic demands.

## Integration

Traditionally, pharmaceutical companies have operated in a very fo-cused manner. While many have both prescription and OTC businesses, they derive the bulk of their sales and earnings from only one segment; a number of companies have diagnostic and equipment interests that are run separately from the core drug business; only in a very few isolated cases are pharmaceutical companies concerned with more than selling to third parties.

Industry integration is favored by several issues:

- There is a blurring of the market place created by government at-tempts to shift costs to patients and by the pharmaceutical indus-try's efforts to prolong the earning potential of brands. Companies now need to manage the life cycle from prescription through to OTC marketing as well as make provisions for controlled generi-cism of their products.
- The convergence of both health care approaches and technology is creating the need for a broader approach to integrated sets of cus-tomer solutions. Health care insurers are beginning to favor early detection, diagnosis, and preventative care as the way to reduce the

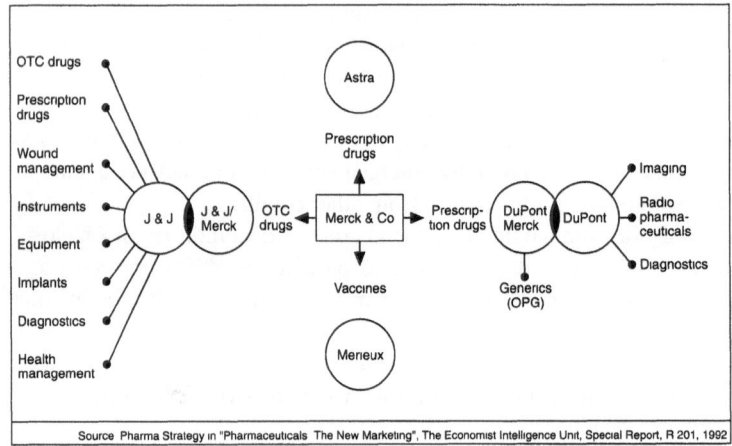

**Fig. 5.** Merck and Co.'s *keiretsu* approach to providing broad integrated sets of customer solutions (from James 1992)

higher costs of treatment; at the same time, a number of advances in diagnostic technology have significant application in treatment.

–   Changes in the channel structure are altering the manufacturer's power in the pharmaceutical market in the industrial world. Concentration in the wholesaler sector and the growth in pharmacy chains are driving the need to obtain greater leverage to offset the new power basis in the channel structure.

Since no company possesses the cash, technology, and skills to operate in such depth and breadth, cooperative arrangements including joint ventures are the preferred route for integration.

The model for an integrated approach to the market is the Japanese *keiretsu* – interlocking mutually supportive groups of suppliers with similar interests. The current role model is the Merck & Co approach (Fig. 5).

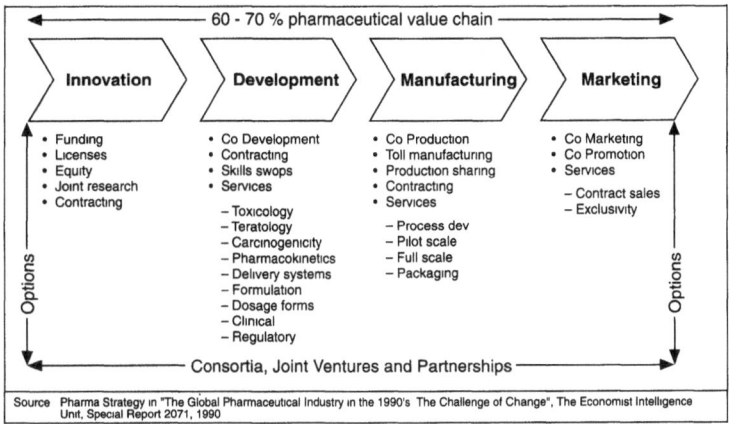

**Fig. 6.** Decoupling the fixed system and outsourcing activities to overcome built-in obstructions to creating value through the pharmaceutical value chain (from James 1990)

## Devolution

There is no longer any part of the process – from funding creative new ideas based on advanced technology, through to the physical marketing of the finished product – where the extra weight of an integrated organization structure is a decisive factor.

Industry devolution is favored by one key new issue: Virtually every functional activity within the pharmaceutical industry can now be contracted out or developed with other companies in strategic alliances. A wide range of high-quality external services (including sophisticated functions ranging from toxicology, carcinogenicity, and teratology to delivery systems and dosage and formulation development; clinical trials and regulatory preparation and submission; pilot plant and full-scale manufacturing; and physical marketing) are now available in many national markets and even globally (Fig. 6).

Devolution provides the opportunity to overcome the widely fluctuating demand for specialist skills by building flexibility into fixed cost structures, helping to move ideas faster and more cheaply from concept to market.

Virtually all companies have begun to devolve functions – buying-in and renting out services to maximize their asset bases. The current industrial model for devolution is the computer industry, in which large companies have been outmanoeuvred by their smaller, more flexible rivals.

## A "Best Guess" Picture of 2010

The structure of the pharmaceutical industry in 2010 will depend largely on corporate responses to the forces driving change within the industry's environment in the mid-1990s. The power and diversity of the trends in the core driving forces – health care delivery, customers, technology, competition, and market structure – are so diverse that no single industry model is likely to emerge (see definitions at end of this chapter). Rather, the structure most likely to be seen is a hybrid, combining elements of concentration, integration, and devolution. This view is based on the following:

- Probably one or two acquisitions and mergers will take place among large and medium-sized companies in an attempt to equal the perceived competitive mass of existing mega-companies.
- The large majority of mergers and acquisitions will take place among multinational, regional, and therapeutic specialists attempting to leverage position through consolidation. This will be driven by the need to gain access to technology and markets and to build defenses against competition.
- Given the costs of acquiring and developing new technology, multi-country firms are likely to be halved in number; those that do not survive will either dissolve into regional or therapeutic specialists or, by acquisition or by being acquired, become multinational companies.
- The growing sophistication of technology and market networks suggests that therapeutic and regional specialists will be able to use proprietary knowledge and in-depth skills to secure sustainable business niches concentrated on high-volume, high-priced market segments.

| | Tier 1 | Consolidations Japanese internationalisation | | Tier 4 (new entrants) | Integrated supply chains |
|---|---|---|---|---|---|
| | | Tier 2 (new entrants) | Tier 3 | | Tier 5 |
| Size ($ bn) | 12 - 14 | 6 - 8 | 2 - 3 | 1 - 3 | > 0.2 |
| Structure | | | | | |
| – integrated | Full | Full | Full | Partial | Limited |
| – decentralised | Yes | Partial | No | No | No |
| Business focus | Broad therapeutic | Broad therapeutic | Therapeutic specialisation | Broad therapeutic | Local supply |
| Market focus | | | | | |
| – private | Yes | Yes | Yes | Yes | No |
| – public | Yes | Yes | Yes | Yes | Yes |
| – commodity | No | Some | No | Yes | Yes |
| Geographic focus | Global | Multinational | Multi-country | Selective | Domestic |
| Innovative spend ($ bn) | 1.2/1.5 | 0.75/1.0 | 0.2/1.0 | 0.2 | > 0.02 |
| – focused (%) | 80 | 100 | 100 | 100 | 100 |
| – prospective (%) | 20 | – | – | – | – |
| Type of innovation | New product | New product | New product | Dosage/ formulation | Regulatory |
| Product differentiation | High | High | High | Medium | Low |
| Profitability | High | High | High | Medium | Low |
| No of firms | 5 | 10 | 10 | 20 | 400 - 500 |

Source  Pharma Strategy in "The Global Pharmaceutical Industry in the 1990's  The Challenge of Change", The Economist Intelligence Unit, Special Report 2071, 1990

**Fig. 7.** The pharmaceutical industry structure, 2010 (from James 1990)

- The real change will come at the national level. Intense competitive pressures and margin compression will eliminate the vast number of largely family owned firms.
- Large national generic manufacturers will emerge in most countries to supply the demand for commodities. Focused generic companies, often linked to larger companies, will create a branded generic segment supplying value-added products and services to specialist markets to command higher margins.
- Despite declining barriers to entry, it will be virtually impossible for a start-up company to become anything but a national boutique.
- The trend towards strategic alliances at all company size levels will continue primarily to obtain skills, technology, and geographic coverage and to provide access to a broad prevention, diagnosis, and treatment portfolio. This will serve to blur the traditional boundaries between companies.
- The traditional organization barriers between the prescription and OTC businesses will disappear as companies begin to adopt life-cycle management, which requires an integrated approach to development and marketing.

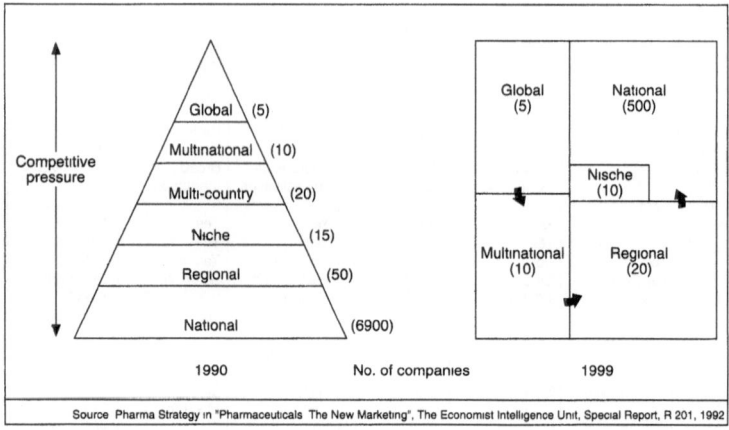

**Fig. 8.** The coming shake-out may lead to a new style pharmaceutical industry with more powerful players operating in more closely defined business segments (from James 1992)

- In an attempt to blunt the power of a more concentrated supply chain, pharmaceutical companies will attempt to forge strong linkages with wholesalers and pharmacy chains, which will involve both formal and informal alliances.
- The demand for flexibility to minimize the fixed-cost base will encourage the expansion of specialist functional suppliers, and one or two companies may evolve into holding companies, contracting out development and brokering marketing rights.

Figure 7 provides an overview of the best guess scenario in terms of industry structure in 2010, and Fig. 8 illustrates the possible new industry shape.

## Appendix: Definitions

*Global:* Operating world-wide with more than 30 wholly owned integrated global production and marketing units and major development units located within the three blocs of the Triad with the capability to develop new products fully (currently Bayer, Hoechst).

*Multinational:* Integrated production and selling units in up to 30 countries with two major product development operations within the Triad (Merck AG, Boehringer Ingelheim, Schering AG).

*Multicountry:* Integrated production and selling units in up to 20 countries with one or two satellite units working on product adaptation (dosage and formulation) in addition to a core home country unit with full product development capability (Boehringer Mannheim).

*Therapeutic Specialists:* Selective operations in up to 10 countries with little or no development capability outside the home country (Fresenius, Immuno).

*Regional Specialists:* Operations in up to five countries with their own production and sales units and with limited product development capability (Asta, Byk-Gulden, Gruenenthal, Luitpold, Schwarz).

*National Companies:* Operating domestically, supplying local markets with repackaged and reformulated products (Madaus, Ratiopharma, Stada, TAD, Wolff).

## References

James BG (1990) The global pharmaceutical industry in the 1990's: the challenge of change. Economist Intelligence Unit, London (special report 2071)

James BG (1992) Pharmaceuticals: the new marketing. Economist Intelligence Unit, London (special report R201)

# 5 Pharmaceuticals and Health Care in Japan Through 2010

Yoshio Yano

To understand the future of pharmaceuticals and health care in Japan, it is necessary to review current trends, to understand not only differences in systems, customs, and culture, but also the procedures used to reach conclusions and decisions. Thus this report is divided into three parts:

1. The health care environment in Japan
2. New product development and the Japanese pharmaceutical industry
3. Foreign drug manufacturers

## The Health Care Environment Through 2010 in Japan

The plausible forecast here is that health care in Japan will still be in good shape by the year 2000 and even by 2010 in spite of several frictions that may emerge among the Ministry of Health and Welfare (MHW), health insurance associations, and health care suppliers. The barometers of health care, such as average life expectancy, infant mortality, etc. (Table 1) are expected to improve even further by early in the next century.

One very significant feature is the balanced increase in health care costs. The growth rate of national health care expenditures per year was around 4%–5% in the late 1980s and is expected to be 6%–7% in the 1990s and 6%–8% in the early 2000s. Health care costs as a percentage

**Table 1.** Health care barometers of major countries (1989)(from OECD)

| Country | Average life expectancy | | Infant mortality | Ratio of national health care to GNP | Per capita health care expenditure | Number of doctors per 10 000 population |
|---------|------|--------|------|------|------|------|
|  | Male | Female | (‰) | (%) |  |  |
| Japan | 75.9 | 81.8 | 4.6 | 6.7 | $ 1035 | 16 |
| Germany | 71.8[a] | 78.4 | 7.5 | 8.2 | $ 1232 | 30 |
| USA | 71.5 | 78.5 | 9.7 | 11.7 | $ 2354 | 23 |
| UK | 72.4[a] | 78.1 | 8.4 | 5.8 | $  836 | 14 |
| France | 72.4 | 80.6 | 7.5 | 8.8 | $ 1274 | 30 |

GNP, gross national product.
[a]In 1988.

**Table 2.** Estimated forecast for national health care cost increase rate in Japan

|  | 1989 (%) | 1990 (%) | 2000 (%) | 2010 (%) |
|---|------|------|------|------|
| Growth rate/year health care expenditure | 5.2 | 4.6 | 6.0–7.0 | 6.0–8.0 |
| Growth rate/year health care expenditure for aged people | 7.9 | 6.0 | 7.0–8.0 | 7.0–8.0 |
| Growth rate/year GNP | 7.2 | 7.6 | 4.0–5.5 | 4.5–5.5 |
| Health care costs as percentage of GNP | 6.7 | 6.6 | 8.5–9 | 10–12 |

Extrapolated from data from the Ministry of Health and Welfare by International Pharma Consulting, Tokyo.
GNP, gross national product.

of gross national product are expected to be around 9% in 2000 and 10%–12% in 2010, according to extrapolations of data from MHW (Table 2). Compared with France, Germany, and the United States, the situation in Japan will be very advantageous (Table 3).

The small increases in health care costs in Japan in recent years can be traced to several factors. Three structural causes are: the small portion of the population that is elderly; the balanced meals eaten by people

**Table 3.** Comparison of estimated national health care expenditure/GNP ratio

| Country | 1987 (%) | 2000 (%) | 2010 (%) |
|---|---|---|---|
| United States | 11.2 | 16–17 | 18–20 |
| France | 8.6 | 11–12 | 13–15 |
| Germany | 8.1 | 10–11 | 13–15 |
| Japan | 6.8 | 8.5-9 | 10–12 |

Data from Health Care Authority of countries concerned from 1987. Estimates for 2000 and 2010 by International Pharma Consulting, Tokyo.

**Table 4.** Trends in reimbursement price cuts of drugs and increase in medical fee in recent years in Japan

| Fiscal year | Medical fee increase (Nominal) | Reimbursement price of drugs | | Net medical fee increase (%) |
|---|---|---|---|---|
| | | Decrease (%) | Equivalent in medical fee basis (%) | |
| | (A) | | (B) | (A)–(B) |
| 1981 | 8.1 | 18.6 | –6.1 | 2.0 |
| 1983 | 0.3 | 4.9 | –1.5 | –1.2 |
| 1984 | 2.8 | 16.6 | –5.1 | –2.3 |
| 1985 | 3.3 | 6.0 | –1.9 | –1.4 |
| 1986 | 2.3 | 5.1 | –1.5 | 0.8 |
| 1988 | 3.4 | 10.2 | –2.9 | 0.5 |
| 1990 | 3.7 | 9.2 | –2.7 | 1.0 |
| 1992 | 5.0 | 8.1 | –2.5 | 2.5 |

Data from the Japanese Ministry of Health and Welfare.

in general; and the easy access to medical institutions, so that diseases are treated in their early stages. Several cost-saving measures taken by MHW have also kept costs down: continued reimbursement price cuts for drugs; strict checks on health care reimbursement claims; and small medical fee increases. Although the share of the population that is elderly is expected to increase early in the next century, this will have fewer adverse effects on health care in Japan than might be imagined, due to the expected drastic shift in policies by MHW.

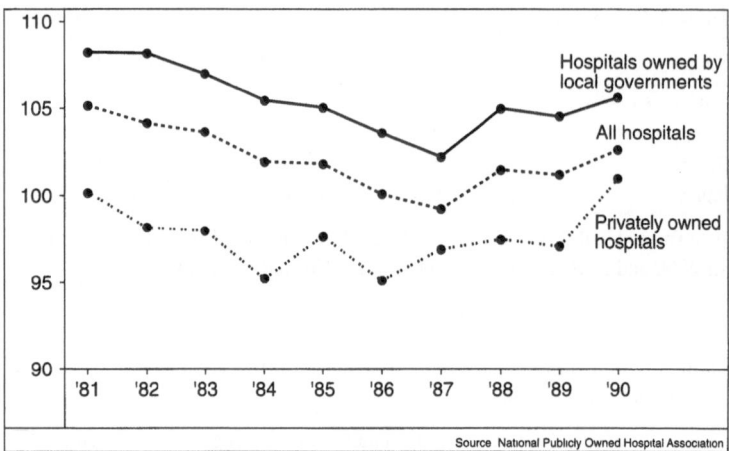

**Fig. 1.** Trends in cost/revenue ratio of hospitals in Japan in recent years (100 signifies break-even point and more than 100 a loss)

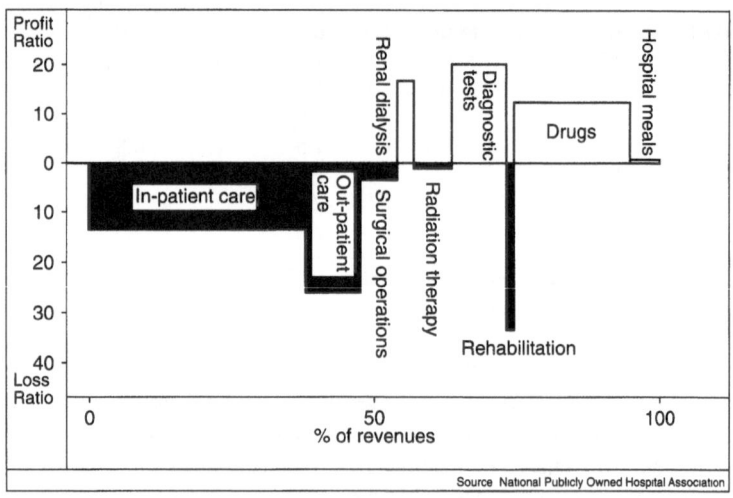

**Fig. 2.** Profits/loss picture of general hospitals by sector in 1990

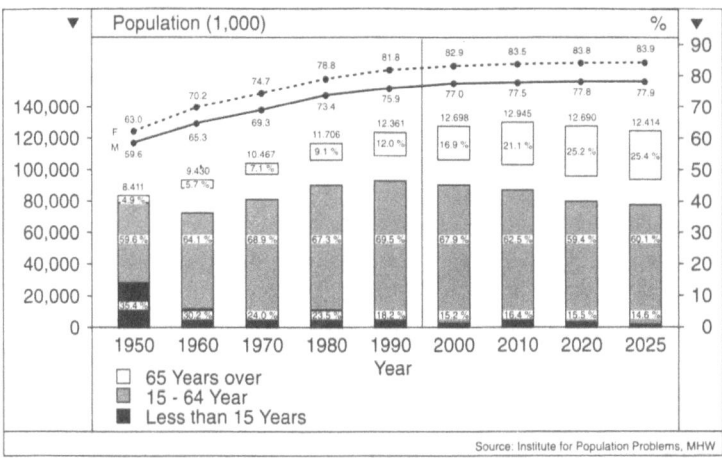

**Fig. 3.** Trends in estimated share by age group among total population towards 2020 in Japan

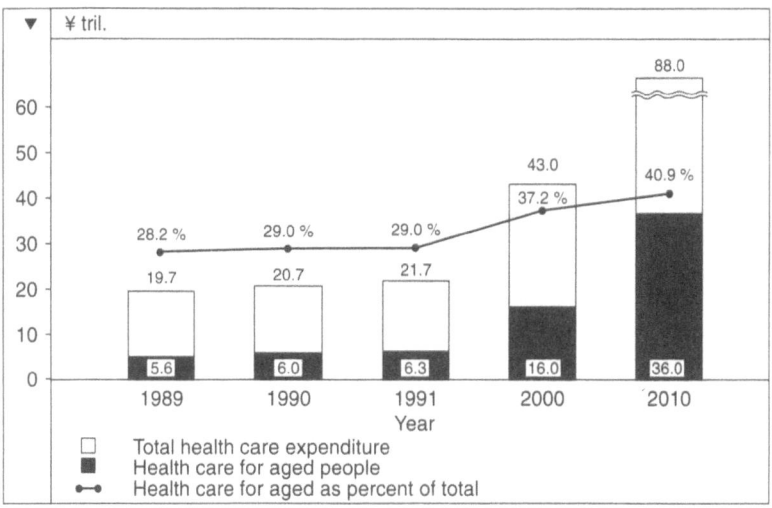

**Fig. 4.** Swelling Health Care Expenditure for Aged People in Japan

**Table 5.** Hypothetical forecast for future Japanese health care expenditure breaking down by category of health care suppliers (unit percent)

| Category | 1989 | 2000 | 2010 |
|---|---|---|---|
| Hospitals | 48.7 | 40.0 | 35.0 |
| Including drug profits | (59.7) | | |
| General practitioners | 21.2 | 25.0 | 27.0 |
| Including drug profits | (27.8) | | |
| Dentists | 9.2 | 10.0 | 10.0 |
| Including drug profits | (9.9) | | |
| Nursing care facilities | 0.1 | 10.0 | 15.0 |
| Drugs | 20.8 | 15.0 | 13.0 |
| Including profits obtained | $(28.7)^a$ | | |
| by medical institutions | | | |
| Total | 100.0 | 100.0 | 100.0 |

Data for 1989 data were taken from National Health Care Expenditure by MHW; future estimation by International Pharma Consulting, Tokyo.
[a]*Bungyo*'s rate may be 20%–25% in the future.

Some of these recent developments can be illustrated. For example, Table 4 indicates the drastic cuts on the reimbursement price of drugs, which are and will continue to be converted to medical fee increases. Second, Fig. 1 documents the financial deterioration of hospitals in the 1980s, which has pushed them to seek drug profits for the compensation of low medical fees (Fig. 2). This is one of the most controversial issues among medical institutions, drug wholesalers, manufacturers, and the regulatory authority. New drug price and distribution regulations are expected to provide remedies for this situation.

Nevertheless, the share of older people in the population will surely increase until 2010–25 (Fig. 3), as will health care expenditures for this group (Fig. 4). Yet these increases will be modified by changes in MHW health care policies such as unit medical fees for care of aged people, a shift of care needing less medical treatment from hospitals to nursing care facilities or home care, and other changes that will be discussed later in this chapter.

Several other notable features of Japanese health care through 2010 can be mentioned. Big changes will emerge in the hospital sector.

Hospitals will only be involved in the treatment of acute or serious sicknesses, the share of which among total health care expenditures will decrease from 48.7% in 1989 to 40% in 2000 and to 35% in 2010 (Table 5). The biggest increase will occur in the category of nursing care facilities, from 0.1% of health care expenditures in 1989 to 10% in 2000 and to 15% in 2010.

The drug sector's share of health care expenditures (excluding profits taken by medical institutions) is expected to drop from 20.8% to 15% by 2000 and to 13% by 2010, a level about the same as in most European nations. *Bungyo* (a health plan in which doctors prescribe and community pharmacies dispense) may lead to a reduction in the drug sector's share including the profits of medical institutions and physicians from 28.7% to no more than 20%–25% of drugs dispensed (in number). The share of expenditures claimed by general practitioners (GPs) will increase slightly by 2010, while that of dentists will change little.

Which aspects of health care cost containment in the years 2000–2010 will mainly be responsible for bringing about these changes? The first is the introduction of unit-based medical fees similar to such fees used for various diagnostic-related services, some of which have already been incorporated for several years. New unit medical fees for chronic-care hospitals rather than acute medical treatment are going to be introduced in April 1993, and other unit medical fees will be gradually expanded to include chronic diseases such as hypertension. This should reduce drug usage by at least 60%.

The second factor is the shift from hospitals to nursing care facilities and to home care, a change encouraged by the generous new medical fees established by MHW in order to get doctors to follow this trend. MHW, in collaboration with the Finance Ministry, is also preparing to transfer the burden of nonmedical care for the elderly from health insurance to accumulated large pension funds in order to alleviate pressures on health insurance schemes.

A third factor is the shift of resources from the drug sector to the medical fee sector, as described earlier. The fourth is that, as in other western nations, patients will increasingly be using co-payments. And finally, MHW's ability to balance the health care budget by 2010 will be the result of a big shift of resources to voluntary private insurance, which will be described later in this chapter.

**Table 6.** Future forecast for *Bungyo* (doctor's prescription): estimated rates of increase in *Bungyo's* share of prescriptions given and their costs

| Year | Prescriptions given (%) | Costs (%) |
|------|-------------------------|-----------|
| 1990 | +12 | +5 |
| 2000 | +20 | +10 |
| 2010 | +25–30 | +12–15 |

Data from MHW and International Pharma Consulting, Tokyo.

The future of *Bungyo* is one issue that is in question. The present ratio – 12% of number of prescriptions and 5% in amount – will increase, but not as fast as expected (Table 6). Even leading officials are forecasting a slow increase in the dispensing of drugs by physicians. This is due to GPs' ignorance about *Bungyo* and the inconvenience of the system for patients compared with the current one-time prescription/dispensing system. In addition, drug profits compensate the physician for low medical fees at the moment. Furthermore, MHW has directed its efforts to encourage *Bungyo* at hospitals instead of at GP practices, because of the GPs' strong opposition, even though only 45% of out-patient care is given in hospitals, compared with 55% given by GPs. Yet MHW influence extends mainly to government-owned hospitals, which account for just 1.6% of out-patient care. Basically, it is ridiculous that the government targets hospitals instead of GPs in its efforts to increase the use of *Bungyo*.

What about the future of the generic market, which is a serious problem area in western nations? Generics now hold 5%–6% of the market and this figure is expected to reach 8%–10% by 2000 and only 15%–20% by 2010. Generics have a negative image among doctors, consumers, and regulatory authorities, which recognize the importance of staying competitive in research and development (R&D) worldwide.

MHW believes that double-decked health insurance (Table 7) will be the extra push that may be needed to balance the health care budget in the late 1990s or early 2000s if the shift of resources from the drug sector to the medical fee sector reaches its limit. This idea springs from the current pension system, in which self-employed individuals can buy voluntary pension insurance in order to receive pensions after age 65 that will compare favorably with those received by company em-

**Table 7.** Double-decked health insurance which MHW intends to introduce during the latter part of the 1990s

| Type of insurance | |
| --- | --- |
| Voluntary | No subsidies but premiums are tax deductable |
| Compulsory | Financed partly by subsidies |
| Voluntary[a] | Health insurance operated by private health insurance company |
| | – National (regional) health insurance for self-employed |
| | – Health insurance for company employed |

[a]There is almost no private health insurance at present in Japan.

ployees. The interesting point here is that self-employed individuals can deduct the premiums they pay from their taxable income up to 900 000 Yen per year, and the government does not pay subsidies on this portion of the pension scheme. MHW and the Finance Ministry intend to transplant this system into health care sometime early in the next decade.

In conclusion, the fundamental health statistics in Japan – such as life expectancy–will continue to improve, and national health care expenditures will maintain balance through 2000–2010, although this may require considerable changes and sacrifices by health care suppliers. Total health care expenditures will increase 6%–7% per year, or at most 8%, through 2000 and beyond, while the pharmaceutical market will grow 2%–4% per year.

The care previously given by many small hospitals and GPs will switch to nursing care facilities, day care, or home care services. Pharmaceutical products that provide therapeutic advances or extra convenience for consumers will register high growth, while those that just imitate other products will not. Thus the products or services that will enjoy significant growth are efficacious drug products, home care services, nursing care services, rehabilitation services, over-the-counter products, membership in health care clubs that provide periodic health checkups, and 24-h telephone services. The federation of MHW and the Ministry of Finance has more power over health care in Japan than is the case in other western nations, it should be noted, because consumers have more in common with what MHW says than what health care suppliers and political parties say. Medical care suppliers and political parties were more closely linked during the days of the late "godfather" Dr. Takemi, former chairman of the JMA.

## New Product Development
## and the Japanese Pharmaceutical Industry Through 2010

What is the R&D capability of the Japanese pharmaceutical industry, and what is it likely to become? First, new product development has improved significantly over the last 11 years, during which Japan has been tied with the United States for the first or second position in the world (Table 8). The quality of Japanese products has also been improving. Japanese companies tied with the Swiss for the number 4 position among the 50 top-selling products in the world in 1990 (Table 9).

For three products – Diltiazem of Tanabe, Lovastatin of Sankyo and G-CSF of Chugai – the second Japanese manufacturer has the worldwide patent rights, except for rights to Lovastatin in the United States (Table 10). (Although Chugai developed G-CSF first, it conceded its patent right in the United States according to the nonpriority rule given to foreign applicants under the U.S. patent law.) Seven promising products are now under development by Japanese manufacturers: Pravastatin, CS-045, YM-175, Epalrestat, FK-506, Levofloxacin, and Sparfloxacin (Table 11).

**Table 8.** Number of NCEs introduced to world market by country of origin 1981–1991

| Country | 1981 | 1982 | 1983 | 1984 | 1985 | 1986 | 1987 | 1988 | 1989 | 1990 | 1991 | Total | Share (%) |
|---|---|---|---|---|---|---|---|---|---|---|---|---|---|
| Japan | 15 | 9 | 10 | 12 | 14 | 15 | 17 | 16 | 9 | 10.5 | 12 | 139.5 | 26.2 |
| USA | 11 | 9 | 9.5 | 6 | 19 | 15 | 13 | 16 | 9 | 9.5 | 13 | 130 | 24.4 |
| UK | 3 | – | 0.5 | 2 | 3 | 3 | 4 | 2 | 3 | 6 | 4 | 30.5 | 5.7 |
| France | 3 | 5 | 3 | 5 | 4 | 2 | 6 | 10 | 2 | 1 | 2 | 43 | 8.1 |
| Germany | 8 | 1 | 9 | 1 | 4 | 5 | 1 | 3 | 3 | 3 | 3 | 41 | 7.7 |
| Italy | 9 | 1 | 1 | 5 | 5 | 2 | 4 | 5 | – | 1 | 1 | 34 | 6.4 |
| Switzerland | 7 | 6 | 6 | 6 | 1 | 3 | 6 | 5 | 3 | 5 | 4 | 44 | 8.3 |
| Spain | 3 | 4 | 1 | – | 4 | – | – | – | – | 4 | – | 13 | 2.4 |
| Netherlands | 1 | 2 | – | – | – | – | – | 4 | 5 | – | – | 6 | 1.1 |
| Sweden | 2 | 1 | 1 | – | 1 | – | – | 3 | 1 | 2 | – | 11 | 2.1 |
| Others | 3 | 3 | 1 | 2 | 1 | 2 | 9 | 11 | 3 | 1 | 4 | 40 | 7.5 |
| Total | 65 | 39 | 40 | 37 | 53 | 47 | 58 | 72 | 35 | 43 | 43 | 532 | 100 |

Unpublished data from International Pharma Consulting, Tokyo.

**Table 9.** Number of top 50 products by country of origin in 1990

| Country | Products (n) |
|---|---|
| USA | 16 |
| UK | 13 |
| Germany | 7 |
| Switzerland | 4 |
| Japan | 4[a] |
| Sweden | 3 |
| Norway | 1 |
| Total | 48[b] |

[a]Diltiazem, Famotidine, Ofloxacin, Nicardipine.
[b]Two products were counted by two different makers each.
(Source: Barclays de Zoete Wedd)

**Table 10.** Innovative NCEs among top 50 products by country of origin in 1990

| Country | n | Product |
|---|---|---|
| USA | 5 | Captpril, Lovastatin, human insulin, EPO, G-CSF |
| UK | 2 | Acyclovir, Intal |
| Germany | 1 | Nifedipine |
| Switzerland | 1 | Cyclosporin |
| Norway | 1 | Johexol |
| Japan | 3 | Diltiazem, (Lovastatin), G-CSF |

Unpublished data from International Pharma Consulting, Tokyo.

**Table 11.** Promising new products under development by Japanese manufacturers in recent years

| Product | Manufacturer | Description |
|---|---|---|
| Pravastalin | Sankyo | Hypolipemic |
| CS-045 | Sankyo | Antidiabetic |
| YM-175 | Yamanouchi | Osteoporosis therapy |
| Epalrestat | Ono | Antidiabetic |
| FK-506 | Fujisawa | Immunosuppresant |
| Levofloxacin | Daiichi | Quinolone anti-infective |
| Sparfloxacin | Dainippon | Quinolone anti-infective |

Unpublished data from International Pharma Consulting, Tokyo.

**Table 12.** Comparison of new high technology products for the future among Japan, Europe and the United States

| Research category | Japan | Europe | United States |
|---|---|---|---|
| Aniotensin II ant. | Takeda | Glaxo, ICI | DuPont |
| Renin Inh. | Sankyo | Roche | Abbot, Pfizer |
| Endothelin inh. | Takeda, Fujisawa | NP Roche, Schering | – |
| hANP | Suntory | Hoechst | Scios |
| Potassium opener | Chugai, Kirin, Yoshitomi, G Cross | SKBeecham, EMerck, Rhone-Poulenc | Wyeth |
| HMG CoA inh. | Sankyo | Sandoz, Rhone-Poulenc | Merck Co. |
| Acyltransferase inh. | Yamanouchi | SKBeecham, Rhone-Poulenc | W-Lambert |
| TPA, 2nd TAP | Yamanouchi, Eisai | Beecham | Genentech, G-Inst. (Sterling) |
| Cardiostimulant | (Otsuka) | (ICI) | (Sterling) |
| Lazaroid, SOD | NPKayaku, Ube, Asahi | – | Upjohn, Chiron |
| Aldose red. inh. | Ono, Takeda, Fujisawa | – | Pfizer, Wyeth |
| Glycosidase inh. | Sankyo, Takeda | Bayer | Pfizer |
| EPO | – | – | Amgen |
| G-CSF | Chugai, Kyowa | – | Amgen |
| GM-CSF | Morinaga | – | Immunex, G. Inst. |
| IL-6 | Ajinomoto | – | Serono |
| C hepatitis | Tonen, Eiken | – | Chiron |
| rDNA albumin | G Cross | Delta | Genentech |
| rDNA hemoglobin | – | Delta | Somatogen |
| Flourocarbon | G Cross | – | Alliance |
| Modified hemoglobin | Ajinomoto | – | Quest, Biopure |
| Proton pump inh. | Takeda, Fujisawa | Astra, SKBeecham | – |
| Immunosuppresant | Fujisawa | Sandoz | Bristol |
| Alzheimer | | | |
|  β-Amyloid | TK Metropolitan | – | Athena, Scios |
|  THA | Sumitomo | Hoechst | W-Lambert |
|  Choline esterase | Eisai, Yamanouchi | Sandoz, Mediolanum | DuPont |

**Table 12.** Continued

| Research category | Japan | Europe | United States |
|---|---|---|---|
| NGF | Takeda | – | Regeneron, Synergen |
| TNF | Dainippon | – | Chiron |
| Antiviral | Yamasa | Wellcome, Astra | Syntex |
| Antisense | Ajinomoto | – | Gilead, Isis, Genta |
| Complement inh. | Mitsubishi | – | TCell Sciences |
| Osteoporosis | | | |
| Calcitonin | Toyo | R-P Rorer | – |
| Bisphosphonate | Yamanouchi | Leira, Gentili | P&Gamble |
| BMP | – | – | Genetics Inst. |
| 5HT3 antagonist | – | Glaxo, SKBeecham | – |
| 5HTI antagonist | Yoshitomi | Glaxo | – |
| Antiprostatis | Ono | Pierre Fabre | Merck |
| IL-1 antagonist | Eisai, Taisho | – | Immunex, Pfizer, Synergen |
| *Totals* | | | |
| Innovations | 18 | 13 | 28 |
| Projects involved | 49 | 33 | 46 |

Original or first reported are underlined.
Unpublished data from International Pharma Consulting, Tokyo.

Table 12 compares new high-technology products expected from Japan, Europe, and the United States, most of which may be introduced 6–10 years from now and which may dominate the world market in each therapeutic category. (Several product categories such as AIDS therapies, the prospects of which are dubious, are excluded from the listing.) The United States is projected to be in the strongest position, with 28 innovations expected, followed by Japan with 18. Yet Japan has the largest number of projects involved in the development of these innovative products – 49 compared with 46 for the United States. So the future of bold new products is very volatile, and even top runners may be forced to pull out of the race. Having a larger number of projects involved means a greater possibility of success at market introduction,

**Table 13.** Sales and R&D expenditure of Japanese drug manufacturers in 1991, fiscal year ending March 1992

| Company | Sales (million ¥) | R&D expenditure (million ¥) |
|---|---|---|
| *Major companies* | | |
| Takeda | 560 918 | 59 300 |
| Sankyo | 359 497 | 33 800 |
| Fujisawa | 226 538 | 33 000 |
| Yamanouchi | 225 874 | 30 000 |
| Eisai | 212 990 | 31 000 |
| Daiichi | 185 002 | 25 000 |
| Chugai | 133 251 | 21 500 |
| *Sub-major companies* | | |
| Taisho | 190 168 | 18 200 |
| Dainippon | 113 496 | 11 500 |
| Yoshitomi | 83 239 | 11 700 |
| Ono | 79 344 | 11 300 |
| Green Cross | 76 999 | 10 000 |
| *Medium-sized companies* | | |
| Kaken | 58 165 | 6 500 |
| Mochida | 55 254 | 8 200 |
| NP Shinyaku | 49 327 | 6 500 |
| *Medium-small companies* | | |
| Nikken | 41 180 | 3 200 |
| Toyama | 39 089 | 6 100 |
| Tokyo Tanabe | 31 529 | 4 400 |
| Kissei | 30 283 | 5 200 |
| Nippon Chemiphar | 17 920 | 2 800 |
| Hokuriku | 16 118 | 3 000 |
| Wakamoto | 10 444 | 700 |
| Nippon Iyakuhin | 8 199 | 442 |

Data from official company reports.

however, and Japanese companies may be in an advantageous position even though they do not have Triad marketing organizations.

The next question is how widespread is the use of new medical technologies in Japan? Commercialization of new high-technology products in Japan will almost parallel that in the western nations, and there will be fewer obstacles to market introduction due to the MHW's being willing to permit the clinical use of such technologies to be covered by health insurance. On the other hand, introducing gene therapies and organ transplants into medical practices will be significantly slower in Japan due to cultural and ethical differences. The diffusion of drug delivery system formulations, which bring benefits to patients and are very common in western markets, will accelerate although not as rapidly as in the west. And they will have less impact on the Japanese pharmaceutical market because of the reimbursement prices given to those products.

New product research is becoming almost impossible, with the R&D cost per one new product standing at $230 million in the United States, $150 million in Europe, $80 million for medium-sized companies in Japan, and $125 million for major Japanese manufacturers (although the figures for Japanese R&D do not include capital costs).

Regarding the capability to produce new products, there are five groups of Japanese pharmaceutical manufacturers at the moment: major companies, sub-major companies, medium-sized companies, medium-small companies, and small companies (Table 13). There is no question about the capability of the major companies, and the sub-major and medium-sized companies are becoming able to produce new products in specific therapeutic categories. The problem area, with some exceptions, is the medium-small and small companies.

In other words, a manufacturer's ability to produce new products may be categorized by an R&D expenditure of 10 billion Yen (about $80 million) per new chemical entity, if the rule of inverse relationship between R&D expenditure and emerging new products applies.

The requirements for a medium-sized drug manufacturer in Japan to survive include average annual sales of more than Yen 100 billion ($800 million) and average R&D expenditures of 10 billion Yen, equivalent to 10% of sales. In addition, the company must be experienced in developing at least two to three new products and have 600–800 medical

**Table 14.** Requirements for global-sized pharmaceutical manufacturer

| | |
|---|---|
| 1. Sales | $3000–5000 million (at 1992 prices) |
| 2. R&D expenditures | $ 300–500 million |
| 3. Sales staff | 1000–1500 in United States, Europe and Japan |

There may be industry restructuring/strategic alliances among Japanese phar-maceutical/Japanese nonpharmaceutical/foreign drug manufacturers towards 2000–2010.

representatives who can cover the nationwide market in order to obtain codevelopment and/or licensing agreements.

Given that, manufacturers in 2000–2010 may fall into four groups:

1. Major companies, consisting of domestic drug manufacturers, domestic nonpharmaceutical producers that have newly entered the drug industry, and foreign drug companies
2. Medium-sized drug manufacturers affiliated with major companies
3. Independent medium-sized drug manufacturers targeting niche products and involved just in the domestic market
4. Many small generic manufacturers

The merger or acquisition of companies may emerge early in the next decade in response to severe cost-saving measures and greater difficulty in new product production or acquisition. Hostile takeovers will remain unlikely due to the Japanese belief that the "concession of a company is the last resort." When an owner, chief executive officer, or the major shareholders decide to seek a merger, instead of visiting a merchant bank they usually first contact companies with which they already have reliable and friendly connections or contacts at the highest level of management.

Regarding the future globalization of major Japanese drug manufac-turers, most have moved from the initial stage of simple licensing through stages of joint ventures and the establishment of clinical trial offices and are now in the final two stages – acquiring small foreign companies and establishing their presence through alliances with foreign manufacturers.

What are the keys to the success of such companies? First, they must have new products, which may be possible. Second, they need to have qualified clinical trials and about 1000–1500 medical representatives both in the United States and Europe, neither of which is possible in the foreseeable future. Finally, their top executives need to have international management knowhow, which could take at least another 10 years. So, major Japanese pharmaceutical manufacturers that are aiming for a global presence need to recognize the necessity of critical mass in the latter part of the 1990s. There may be industry restructuring or real strategic alliances among major Japanese pharmaceutical makers, nonpharmaceutical companies, and foreign drug manufacturers (Table 14).

## The Future of Foreign Drug Manufacturers in Japan

Twenty foreign companies are listed among the 90 top-selling drug manufacturers in Japan, distributed as follows: two in the top 20, seven in the second 20, another seven in the next 20, and four in the final 30 companies (Table 15). Table 16 indicates the operating status of the major foreign drug manufacturers in Japan. All companies have subsidiaries, factories, and medical representatives to promote their products. Sales activities are divided into three categories: sales by their own subsidiaries, joint venture companies, and reliance on their Japanese partners. The first of these categories is increasing significantly. A very limited number of foreign companies have their own research facilities in Japan. The trend in the future will be full-fledged qualification among foreign drug makers with their own research activities in Japan.

It is generally said that a drug company must have more than 800 medical representatives in order to cover the full Japanese market, which is the first step for moving away from relying on Japanese partners for sales. Foreign companies have been aggressively increasing the number of representatives in recent years, and most major ones are already have more than the critical mass needed (Table 17). Recently, several major companies began further expansion to more than 1000 medical representatives in order to compete with their Japanese counterparts, a trend that may spread to other foreign manufacturers in the future.

Increasing the number of medical representatives can lead to difficulties, however, if there is not a parallel increase in the number of new

**Table 15.** Top 90 drug manufacturers (drugs only) in 1991 fiscal year in Japan (units: ¥ million)

| Rank | Company | Sales (million ¥) |
|------|---------|-------------------|
| 1 | Takeda | 371.9 |
| 2 | Sankyo | 310.4 |
| 3 | Yamanouchi | 222.0 |
| 4 | Fujisawa | 204.7 |
| 5 | Eisai | 192.1 |
| 6 | Shionogi | 188.7 |
| 7 | Taisho | 175.0 |
| 8 | Sumitomo | 174.4 |
| 9 | Daiichi | 157.7 |
| 10 | Tanabe | 147.5 |
| 11 | Chugai | 131.1 |
| 12 | Otsuka | 125.9 |
| 13 | Kyowa | 121.7 |
| 14 | Banyu | 104.1 |
| 15 | Tsumura | 100.4 |
| 16 | Dainippon | 92.9 |
| 17 | Bayer[a] | 91.2 |
| 18 | Taiho | 83.4 |
| 19 | Ono | 79.3 |
| 20 | Hoechst[a] | 77.1 |
| 21 | Green Cross | 76.9 |
| 22 | Sandoz[a] | 75.3 |
| 23 | Meiji | 69.9 |
| 24 | Pfizer[a] | 61.7 |
| 25 | NP Schering[a] | 59.3 |
| 26 | Yoshitomi | 58.2 |
| 27 | Asahi Chemical | 56.0 |
| 28 | Kowa | 55.7 |
| 29 | Kaken | 51.6 |
| 30 | SS Pharmaceutical | 51.4 |
| 31 | Ciba-Geigy[a] | 50.7 |
| 32 | Mochida | 47.1 |
| 33 | Teijin | 43.7 |
| 34 | Glaxo[a] | 43.2 |
| 35 | Fuso | 42.9 |
| 36 | NP Shinyaku | 41.3 |
| 37 | Santen | 40.4 |

**Table 15.** Continued

| Rank | Company | Sales (million ¥) |
| --- | --- | --- |
| 38 | Kyorin | 39.3 |
| 39 | ICI Pharma[a] | 39.0 |
| 40 | Roche[a] | 38.9 |
| 41 | Sato | 38.7 |
| 42 | Kanebo | 37.3 |
| 43 | Mitsubishi Kasei | 37.3 |
| 44 | Toyama | 36.0 |
| 45 | Hisamitsu | 32.0 |
| 46 | Torii | 31.9 |
| 47 | Lederle[a] | 31.3 |
| 48 | Nikken | 30.4 |
| 49 | Kissei | 30.2 |
| 50 | Boehringer Ingelheim[a] | 39.8 |
| 51 | Upjohn[a] | 28.1 |
| 52 | TK Tanabe | 27.8 |
| 53 | Bristo/Sq.[a] | 27.7 |
| 54 | SKBeecham[a] | 27.1 |
| 55 | Wellcome[a] | 25.2 |
| 56 | Teirumo | 24.2 |
| 57 | Marion Dow[a] | 23.5 |
| 58 | NP Zoki | 23.4 |
| 59 | Kodama | 23.3 |
| 60 | Schering-Plough[a] | 21.3 |
| 61 | Teikoku Hormone | 20.7 |
| 62 | FujiRebio | 19.7 |
| 63 | Eiken Chem. | 18.7 |
| 64 | NP Chemiphar | 17.5 |
| 65 | Boehringer Mannheim[a] | 16.2 |
| 66 | Mitsui | 16.2 |
| 67 | Hokuriu | 16.1 |
| 68 | Roto | 16.0 |
| 69 | Nippo | 16.0 |
| 70 | Maruho | 15.6 |
| 71 | Toa Eiyo | 15.5 |
| 72 | Lion | 15.1 |
| 73 | Teikoku | 14.4 |
| 74 | Sanwa Chemical | 13.7 |
| 75 | NP Seiyaku | 13.2 |

**Table 15.** Continued

| Rank | Company | Sales (million ¥) |
|------|---------|-------------------|
| 76 | Towa Yakuhin | 13.1 |
| 77 | P&G Health Care[a] | 13.0 |
| 78 | Senju Seiyaku | 12.7 |
| 79 | Wakunaga | 12.6 |
| 80 | Sawai | 12.2 |
| 81 | Chemo-Sero-Therap. | 11.7 |
| 82 | Nissui Seiyaku | 11.7 |
| 83 | Maruishi | 11.6 |
| 84 | Wakamoto | 10.3 |
| 85 | Kaigen | 9.3 |
| 86 | Mikasa | 8.5 |
| 87 | Searle[a] | 8.3 |
| 88 | NP Iyayakuhin | 8.0 |
| 89 | Roussel[a] | 8.0 |
| 90 | Tobishi | 6.7 |

[a]Foreign company.
(Source: Drug Magazine)

**Table 16.** Status of foreign drug companies in 1991 fiscal year in Japan

| Ranking | Number of foreign companies among top 90 |
|---------|-------------------------------------------|
| Numbers 1–20 | 2 |
| Numbers 21–40 | 7 |
| Numbers 41–60 | 7 |
| Numbers 61–90 | 4 |
| Total | 20 |

(Source: Calculated from the data by Drug Magazine)

**Table 17.** Comparison of number of medical representatives by company category in Japan

| Category | Representatives *(n)* |
|---|---|
| Top ranked Japanese companies (Takeda, Shionogi) | 1500–1600 |
| Major foreign companies | 1000–1200 |
| Major Japanese companies | 1200–1300 |
| Sub-major Japanese companies | 1000 |
| Sub-major foreign companies | 800–900 |
| Medium-sized Japanese companies | 800–900 |
| (Meiji, Kyowam Dainippon, Ono, etc.) | |
| Medium-sized foreign subsidiaries | 700–800 |
| (ICI, Boehringer-Ingelheim, SKBeecham, etc.) | |
| Other foreign companies | 400–500 |

products. This problem has prompted the development of new strategic alliances in order to have more new products. If the parent company is in trouble through, for example, due to product failures, patent suits, or generic competition, the subsidiary in Japan can also face trouble if it is not financially independent. Several foreign companies may have to pull out of the Japanese market in the future for this reason.

Seven important factors in the management resources matrix of drug manufacturers in Japan can be identified (Fig. 5): research, development, manufacturing, sales (broken down into detail forces and wholesalers), international activities, and corporate identity. Although foreign companies are good in the first three categories, the sales sector is usually a problem area, even though super products such as Tagamet, Enalapril, and so on sell almost automatically.

Foreign drug manufacturers that want to expand their interests in Japan have two alternatives. One is to complement their strong point (new product research) with the sales capabilities of indigenous companies. The other is to collaborate in overseas markets by exchanging the foreign companies' strong position in sales and the Japanese manufacturers' weak sales capability – a geographical exchange, in other words, of products and sales capabilities.

Foreign drug companies, which have a minimal market share in Japan of 1%, are making long-term plans to acquire a 2%–3% share in

| Drug Manufacturers | Research | Development | Manufacturing | Marketing Detailman | Marketing Wholesaler | International Activities | Corporate Identity |
|---|---|---|---|---|---|---|---|
| Indiginous Pharmaceutical Manufacturers | ○ | ○ | ○ | ◎ | ○ | × | ○ |
| Foreign Pharmaceutical Manufacturers | ○ | ◖ → ○ | ○ | ◖ → ○ | ◖ → ○ | ◎ | ◖ |
| Non-Pharmaceutical Manufacturers | ◖ | × | ○ | × | × | ◖ | ◖ |

◎ excellent    ◖ not enough
○ good          × nothing

Source International Pharma Consulting

**Foreign company's competitiveness factors towards the future**

1) New innovative products
2) Number of qualified medical representatives
3) Adaptability to Japanese market and custom
4) Establishment of good corporate image

**Fig. 5.** Management Resources Matrix of Drug Manufacturers in Japan

the market. Several of them may be able to reach the target and become one of the top 10 companies in Japan, although getting there will be a rough journey.

In conclusion, the indispensable requirements for a foreign company's competitiveness in the Japanese market in 2010 are:

– New innovative products
– A sufficient number of qualified medical representatives
– Adaptability to Japanese market and customs
– The establishment of a good corporate image

# 6 The Environment for the Pharmaceutical Industry Through 2010 in Europe, the United States, and Japan: Alternative Futures

Alternative Future Associates in Cooperation with Schering AG

The pharmaceutical industry of 1990 is dramatically larger, more powerful, and more efficient than in 1970. Looking back to 1950, the industry had very little beyond antibiotics to sell. The next two decades are likely to see change that is greater than during the last four. That much change is often hard to imagine.

Change in the pharmaceutical industry will be driven by research breakthroughs, by cost constraints, by the harmonization of Europe and of the Triad (United States, Europe, and Japan), and by a variety of other factors. Given the range of uncertainty on these major factors, an effective technique for better understanding the future is the development of a range of plausible scenarios or alternative futures that define different paths the pharmaceutical industry and its environment might travel over the next 20 years.

Figure 1 illustrates this. Most organizations have an implicit or explicit view with extrapolates the recent past into the future, call this Scenario A in Fig. 1. The future space occupied by Scenario A (the top of the triangle) is much smaller than that defined by a range of plausible futures (Scenarios A,B,C, and D). And there are other possible futures defined by wildcards. Ironically for most people, if asked in 1987 about the likelihood of the Berlin Wall coming down soon, would have estimated it to be possible but not plausible. The point is that the future

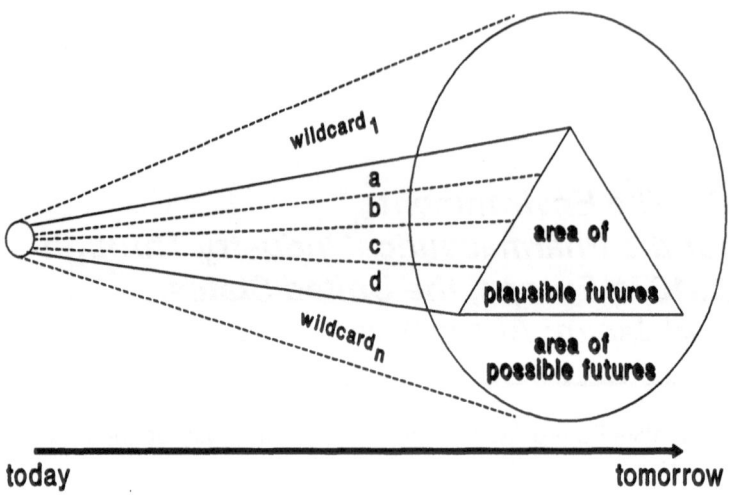

**Fig. 1.** Scenarios: Focus on plausible futures

space for which the company might need to be prepared is larger than is typically considered. Scenarios are a powerful tool for exploring the range of plausible future space.

Take another example where scenarios prepared a company for dealing with an event that other companies were surprised by. The first energy crisis in 1973 caught many oil companies by surprise. Royal Dutch Shell, however, had used scenarios in the early 1970s to prepare the company for a range of possibilities. They were able to use these scenarios to optimize their strategies in the face of the energy crisis and the changes that followed. Scenarios were more widely used in the 1980s. Alternative Future Associates (AFA) has conducted a variety of projects over the decade for the pharmaceutical industry and health care providers, which are not usually published. AFA's parent, the not-for-profit Institute for Alternative Futures, has conducted and published the results of several scenario projects for the pharmacy community, nursing, other health professions, hospitals, the Food and Drug Administation (FDA), and other government agencies (see Appendix).

Scenarios allow a company to explore changes in advance. This is critical in an industry such as pharmaceuticals, where some operating assumptions about the environment are so fundamental that they tend to be ignored. These basic assumptions include the preeminence of the physician in health care delivery and the importance of prescription medications in physicians' armamentarium; the relative absence of price competition among new drug products; the high prices paid for new pharmaceuticals in the United States, Japan, and Germany; and the high research and development (R&D) costs for new drugs. Each of these is likely to change, and the first two are likely to change dramatically.

In addition to considering how a company might address specific challenges in its environment, scenarios also allow the exploration of major internal questions, such as the fundamental question of "what business we are in." Many pharmaceutical companies operate as fine chemical companies with large R&D and marketing efforts. Some think they are in the health business. Such questions will be more pronounced in the years ahead as medical care incorporates richer levels of information, and as consumers and competitors discover the opportunities for health promotion as well as illness care. Thus, for example, the nature of combinations of the physical pharmaceutical product with information or other services may become critical to success. How extensive will the market for such combinations be? Who will pay for them? And how will they affect current modes of pharmaceutical treatment? Scenarios allow companies to explore such questions.

The scenarios in this chapter present four plausible alternatives for the pharmaceutical industry and its environment between now and the year 2010. These images of what might happen will help a company determine what they want to happen and to refine their strategic vision.

Scenarios are important tools for enhancing long-term thinking within a company. They provide strategic intelligence. Their use makes a company smarter. They are "futures for the head." They are pursued in order to make wiser, more effective decisions about what companies want to do in the world. Scenarios help a company better understand how they can shape the future, which must be based on commitments of key individuals throughout the organization and on a shared vision. Commitments come from the heart. Thus in addition to scenarios (plausible futures), companies need to be clear on the vision (their preferred future) of what they are trying to create.

Figure 2 illustrates how scenario and vision related to other aspects of strategic planning. Vision defines where the company wants to go, in

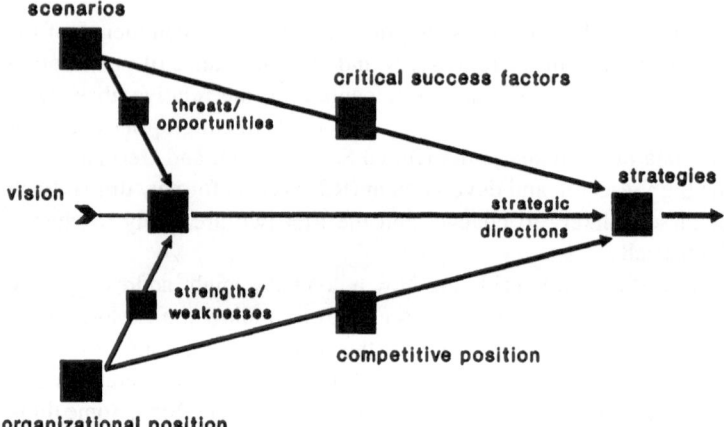

**Fig. 2.** The role of vision

light of the external environment (the top half of Fig. 2). Scenarios identify the threats and opportunities in this external environment. Given the organization's position (the bottom half of Fig. 2), it has certain strengths and weaknesses. Strategies, then, are sets of broad, integrated actions to achieve the vision in light of the external environment (summarized in scenarios) and the organization's strengths and weaknesses.

The scenarios in this chapter represent thematic statements that together present a range of challenges and opportunities. Before identifying the key factors and presenting the scenarios, some caveats are in order. First, for some of the detailed forecasts in the four scenarios, there is more than one "right" or "plausible" answer. For example, cancer breakthroughs might develop in several that would be plausible for that scenario. The scenarios give a sense of the future, but at each juncture several plausible developments could occur.

And finally, the scenarios are not intended to predict the most likely future. Instead, they provide distinctly different environments through which the pharmaceutical industry can identify strategically important opportunities.

The key elements taken as the factors that differentiate these scenarios are the nature or degree of economic development/changes in the pharmaceutical industry, of harmonization within the Triad/general development of the market, of drug research breakthroughs and advances, and of political and legal development/cost effectiveness.

The scenario narratives here weave these elements together differently to create four contrasting stories as seen from the vantage point of two decades hence. The four scenarios are: status quo, the bust, third wave, and frugal and healthy.

## Status Quo Scenario

The Triad economies permitted modest growth in the two decades before 2010, and this period saw the pharmaceutical industry become more mature and stable. High profits permitted both growing R&D expenditures and expensive marketing. The high cost and technical expertise required for new drug development discouraged new entrants despite the attractive return on investment of the existing successful pharmaceutical companies. Markets remained stable while therapies continued to advance with a number of breakthrough products, although not a large number.

Despite periodic weakness in its various economies, the Triad provided a stable environment for business. In Europe, unemployment remained troublesome despite the free movement of labor after 1992. Unemployment was less of a problem in the United States and Japan, but the massive U.S. debt of the 1980s left a weakened dollar that strained economic relations. The threatened collapse of the dollar never occurred due to effective cooperation that stabilized currencies.

During the 1990s, several European countries joined the European Commuity (EC). The United States dramatically reduced its presence in Europe, and Japan joined the peacekeeping forces in exchange for a seat on the U.N. Security Council.

The pharmaceutical industry continued to be profitable largely because of the strength of the Triad markets. The pharma market expanded over this period due to the growth and aging of the Triad populations, and even more because upgraded products brought increases in sales. Pharmaceutical companies were on the defensive over pricing throughout the period to 2010. This pressure led to reduced prices and profits on new entrants and from multisource products in all markets.

The industry is still able to point to impressive scientific progress, even if they have not created a large number of breakthroughs or made improvements in every therapeutic area. Molecular biologists characterized disease processes such as atherosclerosis, cancer metastases, and the buildup of neurological plaques in Alzheimer disease. This type of research did not always lead to blockbuster drugs. Yet it provided a basis for continued progress in all other major therapeutic areas.

Successful companies increased their research efforts in the 1990s. The first or second versions of important new chemical entities (NCEs) were able to command high prices throughout their patented life, thanks to the evidence that they effectively displaced more expensive treatments. Declines in the major chronic disease burden were balanced by increases in such age-related disorders as senile dementia. Cancer deaths continued to rise, however, as the population aged. Better and earlier diagnosis was coupled with treatments targeted on specific tumor sites. This combination improved the survival rates from cancer significantly after the turn of the century.

The commitment to these therapeutic improvements was the foundation for the success of the top strata of the pharmaceutical industry. Industry analysts and insiders agree that a key factor in R&D success was increasing productivity gains through technology. This includes the robotics and supercomputers that became common in the early 1990s and the X-ray holography, expert systems, and gene sequencers that have been found in laboratories since the mid-1990s.

The cultural differences affecting the practice of medicine in Europe slowed internal European harmonization of regulatory approaches to pharmaceuticals. For the most part, labor, capital, and most goods moved freely over borders within the EC by 2005. Compromises on regulation of pharmaceuticals made it easier to gain approval based on the same clinical data, so drug standards and evaluation were effectively harmonized by the end of the 1990s.

In Japan, pharmaceuticals came under increasing pressure because the government saw its health care spending rise dramatically with the rapid aging of the population. Proposals were made to move patients from hospitals into outpatient settings in order to reduce these costs, but the political power of doctors in Japan limited the ability of the Ministry of Health and Welfare (MHW) to make significant reforms.

In the mid 1990s, the MHW attempted to apply pressures to keep pharmaceutical prices down through negotiations, but rising inpatient costs and doctors' fees led the government to seek even greater leverage. By the late 1990s, Japanese doctors lost their dispensing privileges. In addition, the government increased the level of copayment charges patients had to pay. As a result of these changes, the high proportion of the health care bill spent on pharmaceuticals began to decline in the twenty-first century.

Information technologies had a great impact on health care reimbursement and pharmaceutical marketing. In the United States, large government and health care provider information systems expanded their collection of data during the 1980s. These data were joined by a profusion of private inpatient databases from hospital chains, as well as outpatient databases that were maintained by Health Maintenance Organizations (HMOs) and large group practices. By the turn of the century the cost effectiveness of each intervention could be aggregated for almost all clinical settings in the United States, enhancing better medical care. Similar European systems evolved, largely through the prodding of the health care providers.

For all the changes in Japan, the EC, and the United States, the basic characteristics of the pharmaceutical industry remain the same: the industry still provides high-tech, high-value products that are costly to produce because they result from high-risk R&D. While pressures were brought to bear on pharmaceutical prices, the major markets of the Triad paid generously for new medicines, and this brought continued success to the industry.

## The Bust Scenario

The global recession in the 1990s and the depression in 1997 made the pharmaceutical industry decline. Only a few companies were still able to support R&D when it became increasingly difficult to recoup their investments because governments and third-party payers did not allow or would not reimburse drug prices at a high enough level. Therefore many companies became rooted in the production of generic drugs.

To overcome economic hard times, governments in Europe emphasized the protection of their own economies. These measures, combined with the record lows of the U.S. dollar and the worldwide devaluation, nearly led to a complete breakdown of international business relations. One result of this economic crisis was the bankruptcy of national health services and sick funds throughout Europe. Other countries took drastic measures, but by the late 1990s all the health systems in the EC faced common problems.

The late 1990s saw a large number of mergers and acquisitions among the pharmaceutical companies. Many mid-sized and small companies went bankrupt. The firms that survived did so through mergers and joint ventures, and there were only a few newcomers starting up even after the turn of the century when the economy rebounded. No investors were attracted because capital was in too short supply and the risks of pharmaceutical research were too high.

A number of important new products constituted breakthroughs, but public insurers did not provide them, thus only the wealthiest segments of the Triad populations could receive these treatments.

Drugs were seen as more palliative than curative. This made governments reluctant to allow new drugs on the market, much less reimburse them well, unless the advances were shown to reduce cost.

The industry also received terrible criticism for not finding a cure for AIDS. The incidence of the disease peaked in the late 1990s, but remained at a disturbingly high level thereafter. The industry produced treatments, but no real breakthrough was found. In 2010, no definitive cure or prevention strategy for the disease exists.

The economic instability forced governments to control health care costs. Sick funds were dramatically slashed, but ironically the demand for pharmaceuticals increased with the deteriorating economy. Stringent cost controls throughout the Triad region were applied to minimize expenses for health care. In some European countries, physicians were forced to use restructive drug lists and compulsory substitution to cut costs.

Where the price differences continued to exist, parallel importing kept the major pharmaceutical companies from profits they might otherwise have reaped. Many companies tried to defend their position using high transfer prices. The United Kingdom, however, cracked down on this practice, and it became less popular.

The economic downturn was not as serious in Japan as in other parts of the Triad. Nevertheless, neither the government nor employers could afford the rising costs of health care given the economic problems and the growing number of elderly. In 1995 a governmental resolution forbade doctors in Japan from dispensing drugs in exchange for a high capitation fee for their services. When a coalition between the Japan Socialist Party and the *Komeito* toppled the Liberal Democratic Party in 1997, the doctors' lobby lost power and the capitation fees dropped late that year. By the late 1990s, the government had negotiated lower prices with the industry as well, and cut pharmaceuticals to 20% of Japanese health care costs (from almost 30% in the 1980s). By 2010 pharmaceutical costs dropped even further, to 12%.

An even more drastic change in pricing policies occurred in the United States. The pharmaceutical industry lost a major battle when Congress mandated price controls. Rising Medicare costs throughout the early 1990s were led by price increases for pharmaceuticals. The difference between U.S. drug prices and those paid in foreign markets became a subject of media attention. Finally, in a series of congressional hearings, pharmaceutical executives were called to testify over prices. They were raked over the coals by irate politicians. Congress passed legislation for mandatory pricing controls and the FDA was directed to require that, along with clinical evidence of safety and efficacy, cost-effectiveness data must be submitted before new drug application (NDA) approval. While a few breakthrough drugs were granted a price that could support R&D, many companies without such products were forced to curtail research because of financial problems.

For several years, many drug companies had no clear policy on what therapeutic product groups and geographical areas they wanted to trade in, taking a somewhat haphazard approach. By the late 1990s, the consolidation process changed all that. Some small companies were able to survive by creating niches, either in research, through the use of new technologies, or in marketing in specific therapeutic or geographical areas. The main losers were those caught in the middle. Without sufficient critical mass in R&D, they had few compounds and little experience in negotiating the necessary regulatory hurdles.

In addition, they faced increasing difficulty attracting good researchers.

## The Third Wave Scenario

By 2010, Third Wave countries (formerly called "developed nations," the "First World," or sometimes "Triad countries") all had true postindustrial economies. Although steady economic growth in the 1990s and beyond contributed to the economic transformation, people developed a greater environmental awareness focused on local and global ecosystems, as well as an ethic of shared responsibility for conditions in areas of the world removed from their own. Third Wave politicians in Europe, Japan, and the United States encouraged this new worldview. As Alvin Toffler had forecast 30 years before in his book entitled *The Third Wave*, this truly was a great shift, one nowhere more profound than in the pharmaceutical industry.

Health became the primary interest of Third Wave societies. Popular notions about the meaning of health broadened beyond simple sick/not sick dichotomies. Each individual learned to create a personalized health agenda, and health care companies learned to compete to provide individualized assistance. By the mid-1990s, powerful computers in virtually every Triad home offered home health information systems.

The "electronic health" market grew dramatically because of its rich complexity. Much of this software was purchased by and provided to consumers by health providers and major insurers, who had discovered that these can significantly lower treatment costs.

People's intention was to reach "maximum health". Information programmes combined various different components to create personalized health packages which were transmitted to consumers by all means of electronic network.

The new opportunities made the pharmaceutical industry diversify from their base of prescription and over-the-counter (OTC) drugs to a wide range of health interests. Various new companies picked up the information products and became established. The market shares of the traditional pharmaceutical industry were penetrated by these invaders.

Because the cost of microchips dropped significantly during the 1980s and 1990s, these companies found they could bundle relatively cheap information chips with diagnostics, preventives, treatments, and behavioral-change aids into their product lines. Electronic readers in household computer systems accepted the microchip-embedded information that accompanied products. Not only was compliance with prescription regimens improved, but the information had great appeal to a public looking to obtain more individual control over health.

The move to diversify from pharmaceuticals proved to be important to the industry by the end of the decade because the profits from pharmaceuticals sales flattened by the mid-1990s and then declined. Successful breakthrough products displaced many of the standard therapies of the 1970s and 1980s. Most of the new products were based on an ability to work more effectively at subcellular levels. Many were fully decisive, offering cures rather than palliation. Therefore the markets for "halfway medicines" that were not true cures shrunk, and this was particularly true for cardiovascular and cancer products. However, some of the new breakthroughs were not cheap. And some did require chronic use. But most involved only a single treatment course.

The trend to a healthier life-style did not influence health as such dramatically, but it greatly affected pharmaceutical usage. Pharmaceutical unit growth declined in every Triad market, and while enhancement products maintained robust sales, many disease-oriented treatments fell precipitously out of vogue. Those companies that had not diversified into healthy foods, electronic health services, and the new mode of OTCs were in serious trouble.

Companies that did succeed in the new markets of the 1990s had a common commitment to a specific mission: to provide better health rather than simply products or services. They committed themselves to truly significant research and their scientists would talk about the "nobility" of a research target, the "elegance" of the approach, and the "worthiness" of their products. For these researchers, profits were clearly secondary to their corporate pursuits, yet it was these companies that proved to be most profitable in the first decade of the twenty-first century.

New discoveries in research, such as the knowledge of how our bodies handle drugs because of our genes and the understanding of how the body's chemical factory deals with disease, enlarged the demands regulatory bodies made before a new molecular entity (NME) could be approved for marketing. As the genetic basis of the immune system was characterized after the turn of the century, a growing number of pharmaceuticals had to be customized to an individual's unique biochemistry. This need for customization broke up the large Triad market into an increasing number of niche markets; small, entrepreneurial companies learned to quickly identify and exploit the niches in all the major geographic areas.

When computers allowed individuals to pull together an increasing amount of information about themselves, they routinely monitored behavioral-based factors such as weight, age, diet, stress levels, and their mental or learning states. In the late 1990s the combination of electronic health records and home monitoring of health conditions allowed creation of multimillion person databases over several years.

Regulatory bodies increasingly accepted use of these databases for approvals of therapies for individuals rather than for mass markets. Companies that had successfully learned to incorporate large databases into their business diversified into health information services, some becoming vendors to or partners with consumer electronics and other consumer product companies.

Along with the scientific explanation of why acupuncture and homeopathik treatments were successful, small competitors from the alternative sector of the pharmaceutical industry gained ground. Within only a few years, practices once scorned were successfully established in the market.

Social historians looking back at the explosion of health and human development software in the 1990s note that the market reflected more than technological developments. There was also a shift in values throughout the Triad and beyond. People began to emphasize inward satisfactions and personal growth rather than external expressions of material well-being and income growth. This has been termed the "silent revolution" that affected every aspect of society.

## Frugal and Healthy Scenario

Turbulence was the norm from 1990 to 2010, though there was clear movement over time to new paradigms in economics and values. Econmic downturns and hard times were recurrent. As economies transformed, social and ethnic strife was a major feature not only in Eastern Europe but in all regions of the world. Yet, equally visible as the new civilization emerged were significant value shifts among a majority of individuals in the Triad countries, which redirected economic and technological development. Ecologically and socially sustainable development became the norm in most countries, industrial and developing.

Technological development in the context of these changes and the recurring economic recessions focused increasingly on human needs and environmental consequences. Information technology, for example, offered great capabilities. The recessions only slowed the development of an enhanced form of home telephone service by a few years. This service allowed the transfer of movies, whole encyclopedias, and novels at minimal costs. Communities used these information systems to build better networks, which allowed smarter shopping for all types of products. Doctors, treatments, and hospitals could be compared – just as automobile or appliance repair shops could – by their users on the basis of consumer satisfaction and other outcomes. With more effective data, consumers could link their values to their search for the best products.

Health care, particularly the government-funded or tax-supported systems, became more frugal. Outcomes were used to show the comparative efficacy of various treatments and preventive strategies. These outcome measures also compared the results of various types of providers with those of self-care. Prevention, self-care, lower-cost providers, and therapies were favored.

Also, it was shown that the integration of therapy with low-cost, minimally invasive diagnostic technologies was the most appropriate. The selection of type of therapy to include in frugal, basic health plans became a matter of public discussion and conscious priority setting. More holistic and cost-effffective therapies quickly gained the upper hand. Local and national communications systems allowed information on the relative value of therapies and providers to be quickly communicated. And it allowed regulators to relax the requirements of licensure.

A broad range of practitioners – from nurses and acupuncturists to physicians – practiced on the basis of an initial certification from their specialty. In order to continue practicing, however, they needed to have good patient outcomes. The advanced information systems in place in most countries of the Triad by 2000–2005 gathered and analyzed these outcome data.

In this environment, older pharmaceutical therapies that were still effective became commodities, with commodity margins. Generics became the dominant standard medication when drugs were used. Yet the information systems and outcome measures allowed health care to be customized effectively to individual patients. And standard pills were integrated into packages that included diagnostic components, information sharing, and behavior-reinforcing components. Except for the clearly outstanding generics and a limited number of vaccine-like fully decisive medications, most pharmaceuticals have been integrated into therapeutic packages.

Another surprise was the dramatic reduction in R&D costs. The ability to simulate and automate various aspects of the discovery and development processes through virtual reality meant that cybernated animal and human populations served as test cases for many aspects of drug R&D. This helped lower the number of individuals needed for testing before marketing and to speed the discovery process for many compounds. For drug development, large health care providers through-out industrial countries recognized the value of having ever more potent and cost effective remedies.

The information systems and personal monitoring equipment used by health care providers and their consumers meant that normal medical practice and preventive activities automatically captured more and bet-ter data than the clinical trials of the early 1990s. Large health care providers got into the drug development business directly – sometimes in partnership with pharmaceutical companies, sometimes inde-pendently. These new entrants could easily add information and beha-vior-shaping components to their compounds in their therapies.

Regulators also changed their perspectives. Cooperation among health care providers (the British National Health Service, some of the German *Krankenkassen*, and, in the United States, large HMOs such as Kaiser Permanente), pharmaceutical companies, and regulators to ex-pedite discovery and development led to more rapid and effective test-ing and approval. Given the greater ability to predict likely side effects, to capture, record, and aggregate side effects as they occur, and to incorporate that learning into the expert systems that guide diagnosis and prescribing, regulators were willing to lower the pre-market thre-shold. Together, these changes led to much lower development costs.

While the pharma companies of the early 1990s spent roughly 20% of their sales for various types of marketing aimed at influencing physi-cians' discretion in writing prescriptions, most companies in 2010 spent only 2%–4%. The information systems (physicians, regulators, insurers, and consumer groups) that aggregated outcome data into clinical algo-rithms related to individual patient data – including ability to pay – led to this change. The day of a detail person who visited physicians was over by the late 1990s. When a physician makes a diagnosis, given the conditions of the patient, the appropriate and appropriately cost effective medication is identified for the physician. The resulting elimination of much pharmaceutical sales and marketing efforts contributed to the decline in the cost of pharmaceuticals.

Although there is still a very large market for traditionally manufactured drugs, a significant portion of the pharmaceutical marketplace has shifted to small batch or individually focused production. This led clinical labs – inside and outside of hospitals – and high-tech pharmacies to become the location for much twenty-first century "compounding".

The pharmaceutical industry experienced a "fall from grace" from the mid-1980s through the mid-1990s as their high prices, marketing practices, and slow contribution to breakthroughs led to much public criticism. Coupled with an environment of cost containment, commoditization, and customization, the economic basis of the pharma industry changed dramatically. Market size for specific drugs decreased with therapeutic subgrouping and customization. Cost constraints from health care providers kept pressure on prices. Many companies went under before the new R&D approaches emerged. The companies that remained were often the results of multiple mergers. Also, the most successful companies integrated their drugs with noninvasive or minimally invasive diagnostics, and with information and behavior shaping programs. Many of the remaining pharmaceutical companies merged with food and other consumer product companies.

After the year 2000, given the lower cost of R&D and the health information systems that effectively did the marketing needed, new start-up companies emerged, often developing joint ventures with health care providers who did the testing. The pattern of companies operating in what had been the pharmaceutical therapy arena was far more diverse by 2010. But the industry had also regained its stature. Dramatic breakthroughs occurred often, the side effects of drugs were much better targeted and prevented, companies dramatically lowered their marketing costs, and some companies actually took a leadership role in developing the more integrated and holistic modes of therapies.

# Appendix

### Scenarios for the Pharmacy Community
Bezold C, Halperin JA, et al. (eds) (1986) Pharmacy in the 21st Century. Institute for Alternative Futures and Project Hope, Alexandria, Virgina

### Scenarios for Nursing:
Bezold C, Carlson R (1986) Nursing in the 21st century: an introduction. J
Prof Nurs January-February: 2–8 (see pp. 2–71 for related articles from the
July 1985 Conference on Nursing in the 21st Century)

### Scenarios for Health Professions
Bezold C (1989) The future of health care: implications for the allied health
professions. J Allied Health Fall: 438–457

### Scenarios for Hospitals
Bezold C (1992) Five Futures. Healthcare Forum May/June: 29–42

### Scenarios for Food and Drug Administration
Peck JC, Rabin KH (1989) Regulating change: the regulation of foods, drugs,
medical devices and cosmetics in the 1990s. Food and Drug Law Institute,
Washington DC

### Scenarios for Government Agencies
On the future of health promotion, particularly in the workplace:
Bezold C, Carlson RJ, Peck JC (1986) The future of work and health. Auburn
House, Dover, Massachusetts

## 7  Workshop Summary:
## Change in a Challenging Future

Clement Bezold and Linda Starke

Health care delivery, therapies and pharmaceuticals face major changes throughout the industrial world in the form and delivery of health care. As cost containment strategies are introduced by governments, as payers become more influential in decisions about therapies, and as consumers become more involved in directing their own health care, health care providers and pharmaceutical companies are being challenged to rethink the way they do business. To explore this challenge Schering AG held a workshop in December 1992 which focused on the papers in this volume. This chapter summarizes the discussions at the workshop. This workshop mixed scenario presentations and discussions with the papers developed by leading experts. Together they are intended to give the reader an enhanced sense of what the future holds and the enhanced capacity for more imagination and creativity.

Dr. Clement Bezold of the Institute for Alternative Futures (IAF) and facilitator for the workshop opened with a review of current and long-term trends in the pharmaceutical environment. All industries in the "turbulent 1990s" are in a period of economic uncertainty, with no clear guidance on whether we are fundamentally transforming our economies or are coming out of a recession into a more familiar pattern. Pressures facing pharmaceutical companies include demographic growth and movement, political activism, and the major changes in the form and delivery of health care. Newly available information systems and those on the horizon are one of the forces altering the delivery of health care.

## Health Care Information Systems in 2010

Jonathan Peck of IAF discussed the explosions in automated inpatient information, outpatient information, and health information in homes that will affect the pharmaceutical industry in the next decade and beyond (see Chap. 1). The computers we know today should not be thought of as the models for tomorrow: the power of computers is quadrupling every few years, so when considering the impact of information technology on health care and pharmaceuticals in the future, it is better to be bold in estimates of what computers will contribute.

By the late 1990s, patient information will be fully automated. Doctors will increasingly be tied into computer systems and be using therapeutic information that is customized for particular patients. In the Triad countries (Japan and the European and North American countries) this will be part of a transition from industrial to information-based economies.

New partnerships will arise – with companies that produce expert diagnostic, therapeutic, preventive, and consumer information systems, with doctors who are plugged into them, and with patients themselves. The long-term success of any pharmaceutical company will depend on early recognition of the challenges presented by this next revolution in information systems.

Doctors or pharmacists in the future will consider themselves partners with their patients, able to make home visits, albeit electronically. The technology is going to change dramatically the way information reaches people. By the end of this decade, many homes will be linked into medical networks electronically, and consumers will allow people to monitor the progression of their own conditions and diseases. The patient is going to enter the decision-making arena with much greater information.

A shift in the traditional role of physician as primary decision maker has already occurred as payers become much more important in decisions about appropriate therapies. As information on patients in all settings – inpatient, outpatient, and at home – becomes automated, the pressures of cost containment will increase payers' desires to be full partners.

The pharmaceutical industry is not far behind others in the takeup of emerging information technologies; things are moving very rapidly in some areas, such as field force automation. It is not as far along, however, as the banking industry, for example. This may be a reflection of its historical reliance on a captive audience – doctors. And also due to the fact that once a product is initially approved, there has been little accountability about its use, the public has had little reason to ask for information about it. These factors will change in the years ahead.

Health outcome research is starting to use quality-of-life assessments. For example, in many U.S. hospitals therapeutic selection is checked automatically and any discrepancies with the expected selection are brought to light. Another example of the use of expert systems that is likely to become more common is a joint effort between Harvard Community Health Plan (a health maintenance organization, HMO) and the software and services company EDS that has put computers in patients' homes in an experimental program. This will dramatically enhance the ability of consumers to do self-care at home.

## Pharmaceuticals and Health Care in the Twenty-First Century

Three contributions discussed various aspects of health care and the pharmaceutical industry over the next 20 years. Willis Goldbeck, influential U.S. health policy expert and consultant to WHO Europe and the European Community (EC), discussed the changing shape of the health care field (see Chap. 2). The forces at play include:

- A lack of relation between per capita spending and actual health care outcomes
- Dissatisfaction with current systems in the United States and Europe
- A varying role for physicians
- A growing number of jobs in the health care industry, in all its forms, rather than a contraction, as commonly assumed

Mr. Goldbeck expects more direct contact between pharmaceutical companies and consumers, which already occurs in the form of providing information, and increasing political support for reaching health objectives, as evidenced by the backing for WHO's Health for All

Strategy. The WHO strategies contain broad principles and targets on health policy, health professions and institutions, economics, environment and health, and the role of individual life-styles. Before the Maastricht Treaty is even agreed to by all parties, the EC is considering setting up a Health Directorate, collecting Community-wide information, and collaborating internationally.

Patients are going to demand accountability and know how to use the information collected because of the revolution in computer technologies. He noted that the physician–patient relationship is already changing for many patients, who are becoming more involved in therapy decisions. Mr. Goldbeck, who is directing a major health information systems project for WHO Europe and the EC, agreed with Mr. Peck's assessment of the technological explosions of the next 20 years for the United States and Europe.

By 2010, most successful pharmaceutical firms will not just be drug firms: some will have been acquired by other health care concerns or by information industry companies; others will have done the acquiring. U.S. companies are diversifying in different directions, in part in reaction to public scrutiny of their pricing structures, and this could offset in part any reduction in drug use as life-style changes become a more popular "therapy". Mr. Goldbeck noted that pharmaceutical companies will increasingly act as successful individual companies, not as an industry.

Dr. Louis Lasagna, Director of the Center for the Study of Drug Development at Tufts University, discussed the future of pharmaceutical therapy and regulation (see Chap. 3). Although physicians will still be important prescribers in the future, clinical pharmacists are bound to have a growing role, a trend marketing departments should note. Company representatives will continue to interact with physicians, but they will be talking about the physician's specific needs rather than delivering a lecture on a new product.

Although blockbuster breakthroughs are unlikely in the near term, more modest advances are still terribly important; a palatable liquid version of an antiepileptic, for example, would be a significant advance for treating epileptic children. Dr. Lasagna noted that rationing of health care is inevitable, but by this he does not mean inequitable access to health care – which occurs everywhere and seems unavoidable. Rather, he means having the ability to provide specific therapies but deciding as a society whether we can afford it or not. This will involve painful choices but will occur.

All these decisions on rationing, quality of life, and so on are up to the public, as it is their health and money that is involved. But this does not make the decisions any easier, as the experience with public priority setting in Oregon, USA, has shown. When considering where to cut costs, it is important to remember the cost of not delivering drugs: it may be expedient but may cost more in the long run.

One dilemma concerns the expense of real innovation versus the poor public image of the pharmaceutical industry because of what are seen as high prices. The British approach of controlling profits, not prices, is worth considering. The British penalize companies, for example, that spend too much on advertising. The assumptions this is based on are valid – pharmaceutical companies are good for society, they can contribute to a positive trade balance, and they provide employment. Calculations must be made about how much profitability is required to keep them innovative.

But if profit control is to be supported, so must a profit guarantee or minimum. Some workshop participants felt that profit control, which may happen naturally anyway in the marketplace, is dangerous in the political arena, where it can become just a slogan in the hands of politicians. In no other industry in the world does government step in and say you can make only so much money.

Prevention is one important measure for cost containment. As only rich patients are able to get regular screening today for some costly diseases, there may be a role for industry in developing cheaper screening technologies. A company that came up with a cheap, reliable screen for obesity or colon cancer, for instance, would make a great contribution.

Dr. Lasagna noted that patients need to pay to some extent for health, given its broad definition. How can we bring to the public the message that health cannot be guaranteed and cannot be provided just by government? That the pockets of the public must also be open? Copayments are one answer.

Barrie James of Pharma Strategy Consulting AG in Basel, Switzerland, spoke about the shape of the industry itself (see Chap. 4). The pharmaceutical industry has enjoyed a stable environment over the last 40 years, with buyers who had a relatively low sensitivity to price.

Competition has been based on the ability to find a new drug. This is all changing, and the success of the industry as a whole in the future will depend on how it handles the pressures to reduce the overconsumption of scarce resources, to deal with emerging diseases that are more difficult and expensive to diagnose and treat, to respond to the growing incidence of noncommunicable life-style diseases, and to take various other steps seen as necessary.

As governments began to face the cost crisis, they realized they need to control both supply and demand, so they have tried to affect the decisions of physicians, pharmacists, and patients. Public and private insurers are now in the driver's seat; they can control profits, margins, and market shares. Another big change facing companies is the variety of customers and network of interests they must respond to.

Costs are obviously a big concern. For a pharmaceutical company to be in business focused on general practitioners (GPs) in the eight countries that account for 80% of the profits of the pharmaceutical industry requires a sales force that costs on average $290 million per year. Market competition is becoming fierce. Three possible forces will shape the industry: consolidation, integration, and devolution.

Consolidation among some of the 7000 pharma companies worldwide – with the largest holding a market share of around 5% – may occur through mega mergers and selective acquisitions aimed at strengthening a geographic, product, or technology portfolio. Integration will involve broadening the depth and breadth of a company, covering prescription and over-the-counter (OTC) business, diagnostic and equipment interests, and a fuller scope of marketing arrangements; this is likely to occur through cooperative arrangements with other firms. Devolution can build flexibility into fixed cost structures, as the computer industry has discovered, by contracting out such activities as delivery systems, clinical trials, and formulation development. In the end, noted Mr. James, the future is likely to be a combination of these three elements. In two decades, he expects some 15 countries to account for about 60% of the industry's profits, so from that point of view there will not be a drastic change from the present.

Although the pharma industry has received a large number of blows during the last two decades, these are only now beginning to affect the bottom line. It is the control of both supply and demand that is now proving difficult to surmount. Mr. James defended the trend of consumers wanting to know what treatments are being prescribed and what alternatives exist. Companies cannot just decide to develop a new product and introduce it in the hope that it will be popular; they need to find out what patients want. Glaxo, for example, has done this through focus groups of patients and physicians.

## Pharmaceuticals and Health Care in Japan Through 2010

Professor Yoshio Yano of International Pharma Consulting provided a look at the special situation in Japan now and over the next 20 years (see Chap. 5). Japan is fundamentally similar to other industrial countries, but is also a bit different in culture and the systems used. There is almost no private health insurance, for example. Health care is widely available, but hospitals have been running at a loss since 1987, mainly due to the cost of both inpatient and outpatient care. The drug industry is the biggest source of profits for hospitals. The market for generic drugs, which is growing rapidly in most western nations, is not expected to grow as fast in Japan, reaching perhaps 15%–20% by 2010.

The aging of Japan's population is a matter of great concern: the share of the population over 65 is expected to rise from 12% in 1990 to more than 25% by 2025, with the percentage of health care expenditures for those over 70 rising dramatically from 6% to 36% during the same period. One notable factor affecting health care in the future is the average age of GPs: it is now 60, so most GPs will be retiring in the next 15 years.

Japanese doctors using a system like diagnosis-related groups (DRG) do not alter diagnoses in order to gain higher payments, as apparently has happened in the United States. The Japanese Medical Association is still strong, so it does not seem that the *Bungyo* system (when doctors prescribe and community hospitals and/or pharmacies dispense) will be widely used very quickly.

Professor Yano noted that doctors and pharmaceutical companies are going to suffer together from cost containment.

## Alternative Futures Scenarios

Working groups considered four scenarios for the year 2010 prepared
by Schering and the Institute for Alternative Futures (IAF, see Chap. 6).
Dr. Bezold of IAF noted that scenarios are not predictions of "the"
future, which are not only impossible to make but also counterproduc-
tive. Because the future is uncertain, giving people the impression that a
particular scenario is "the" way the future is going to unfold is not really
helpful. The future contains a variety of possibilities and opportunities;
alternative scenarios are a technique that helps you to be mentally
flexible. They provide a powerful tool for exploring the future in the
face of uncertainty. Working with them in turn permits you to act more
effectively.

The four scenarios considered were:

- *Status quo* – This is basically an extrapolation of the current system,
  with rapid harmonization in Europe of regulatory approaches and
  better therapeutics, diagnosis, and prevention programs.
- *Bust* – Economic hard times become a major pressure on the pharmaceutical industry, forcing mergers, acquisitions, and failures;
  governments control costs, and high prices for drugs meet strong
  objections in most countries.
- *"Third wave"* – This assumes that a healthy life-style becomes a
  therapy in its own right and that an information revolution permits
  customized therapy from a range of providers; approval of regulatory bodies is speeded up by postmarketing data systems.
- *Frugal and healthy* – In this scenario, the world moves from materi-
  alistic values towards community and quality of life concerns; marketing and research and development (R&D) costs are lowered dramatically, new information systems give consumers more control,
  and pharma markets are customized and integrated.

In considering these four scenarios, it is important to remember that the
pharmaceutical industry is at a watershed, and that the past is not a guide
to the future.

Dr. Bezold also spoke about corporate vision. This can be summarized as the compelling, inspiring statement of what the company
wants to create. A mission is the purpose of an organization, while a

vision is the end point of what the company wants to create. Most companies let circumstances determine their behavior, which then determines their aspirations, albeit limited ones. A vision will create a strategic advantage, particularly in an era of rapid change.

As the pharmaceutical industry faces change in connection with cost containment, the information revolution, consumers and payers determined to be more involved with therapy decisions, and both consolidation and integration, companies that have a vision, remain flexible, and anticipate alternative futures will be much better prepared to succeed. While the workshop participants were not uniform in their support of the need for pharmaceutical companies to use visioning to reinvent themselves, many felt this was essential.

The discussions using the scenarios clearly show that there are some changes the industry is facing that reinforce some of the earlier expert discussion, particularly the links between pharmaceuticals, life-style, other therapies, and outcome measures. The strategy that allows compounds to be developed without very conscious attention to how it can be optimally used in combination with more sophisticated behavior change and life-style therapies, as well as with OTCs, will no longer be successful.

# Subject Index

abortion 31
AIDS 5, 42
AIDS lobby 42
Alternative Future Associates 1, 89
alternative futures 89
alternative therapies 56
American Medical Association 2
analog empire 6
artificial intelligence 9
automated protocols 24
automatic measurement
   of all drug use 34

baby boomers 5
bioavailability 44
biotechnology 29
Bungyo 73

cancer 42
clinical algorithms 102
comparative data systems 35
comping and voice input 16
computer-assisted new drug
   applications 19
consolidation 110
consumer evaluation systems 23
consumer information systems 22
core driving forces 62
corporate vision 112
cost analyses 44
cost containment 5, 106

cost control 33
cost controls 96
cost distribution mechanisms 33
cost effectiveness 95
cost-effectiveness studies 21
cures 42
customization 4

decentralization 4
devolution 61, 110
diagnostic-related groups 4
diagnostic-related services 73
digital networks 17
digitization of data 6
direct broadcast satellites 18
direct nervous system control
   of computers 16
disintermediation 4
distributed computing 12
DNA fingerprints 20
double-decked health insurance 74
drug pricing 45
drug utilization review 25
drugs 33
DUR 5, 25
DUR programmes 25

eastern medicine 37
electronic games 3
environmental disasters 36
ethnic and religious conflicts 37

expert systems   9, 13, 21-22, 94
external environment   92

fine-tune treatment   42
flexible information processing   13
formularies   35
fourth paradigm of computing   7
frugal and healthy scenario   100

gene sequencers   94
gene sequencing   43
generic companies   63
generic drugs   47, 111
generic market   74
GI generation   5
gigaflops   11
global recession   95
globalization of the health care
   industry   34
groupware   9
growth factors   43

Harvard Community Health Plan
   107
health care   67, 75
health care delivery   50
health care in the 21st century   107
health coach   23
health information systems   1
health outcome measures   20
high growth products in Japan   75
holographic displays   17
home health aides   33
home health care   46
hostile takeovers   82
human values   31
humane genome project   29
hybrid architectures   11
hypermedia   9, 14, 34

individually focused production
   103

information revolution   1
information technologies   95
integration   59, 110
integration of mind and body   38
interactive computer systems   42
international data bases   2

joint ventures   82

keys to success   82
knowbot software   18
knowbots   14

language processing   15
leaders   32
licensing   82
life-cycle management   63

machine learning   11
management of innovation   29
management resources matrix
   87-88
market structure   56
mass migration   36
medical practice guidelines   24
medical practice management
   systems   24
mega mergers   58, 110
microcomputers   10
microelectronics   10
microsupercomputers   10
miniaturization   8
mobile communication   17
molecular genetics   43
molecular nanotechnology   29
monitoring systems   25
multimedia communication   7
multimedia devices   8

nanofabrication techniques   10
narrowcasting   15
networking of digital networks   8

neural networks   8, 11
new partnerships   106
new product development   76
new product research   81
nurses   33

open systems architecture   34
optical fiber   8
optical fibers   17
optical storage   15
orphan drugs   48

paradigm shift   6
parallel importing   96
parallel languages   13
parallel processing computer
    architectures   11
patient advocates   42
patient empowerment   5
patient information   106
pattern recohnition   11
personal computers   3
personalized health agenda   98
personalized health packages   98
environment   49, 89, 93, 95
pharmaceuticals   67
– in the 21st century   107
pharmacies   53
physicians   41
plausible futures   90
post-market surveillance   34
post-marketing surveillance   19
prevention   109
prevention of disease   46
price concessions   53
price controls   97
price erosion   56
productivity gains   94

QMR expert system   21

reimbursement   44
research tools   19

scenario-driven analysis
    and planning   30
scenarios   29, 31, 90, 93
scientific progress   94
Single European Act   32
soft logic   14
software   12
space exploration   31
speech recognition   8, 15
spirituality   37
standardized products   52
status quo scenario   93
strategic alliances   61, 63
strategic intelligence   91
strategic planning   30
super-scale integration chips   10
synthesis of computing
    and communication   7

tactical implementation   30
telecommunications   17
teraflops   11
therapeutic packages   102
Third Wave scenario   98
Third World   35
trends   30
tribal conflicts   37

unmet needs   42

value   35
vision   91
visual graphic techniques   43

wholesalers   53

X-ray holography   94